医療系学生のための

つたわる英語 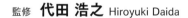Web音声付

English Communication Competency
for Future Healthcare Professionals

監修 **代田 浩之** Hiroyuki Daida

編集 **並木 有希** Yuki Namiki
Marcellus Nealy ニーリー・マーセラス
Tom Kain ケイン・トム

南江堂

監 修

代田　浩之　　　　　順天堂大学保健医療学部　学部長

順天堂大学保健医療学部診療放射線学科　特任教授

順天堂大学大学院医学研究科循環器内科学　特任教授

編 集

並木　有希　　　　　東京家政大学人文学部英語コミュニケーション学科　准教授

Marcellus Nealy　　順天堂大学医学部一般教育　准教授

Tom Kain　　　　　文京学院大学　非常勤講師

執 筆（執筆順）

Marcellus Nealy　　順天堂大学医学部一般教育　准教授

浅野　恵子　　　　　順天堂大学医学部一般教育　教授

Clay Bussinger　　　順天堂大学医学部一般教育　非常勤講師

Deborah Grow　　　順天堂大学医療看護学部一般教育　教育講師

Andrew N Mason　　順天堂大学医学部一般教育　助教

藤田　亮子　　　　　順天堂大学医学部一般教育　准教授

並木　有希　　　　　東京家政大学人文学部英語コミュニケーション学科　准教授

Tom Kain　　　　　文京学院大学　非常勤講師

藤倉　ひとみ　　　　順天堂大学医療看護学部一般教育　助教

大野　直子　　　　　順天堂大学国際教養学部　准教授

編集協力

折田　創　　　　　　順天堂大学医学部上部消化管外科学　准教授

Malcolm V Brock　　ジョンズ・ホプキンズ大学医学部外科学　教授

順天堂大学医学部上部消化管外科学　客員教授

坂野　康昌　　　　　順天堂大学保健医療学部診療放射線学科　特任教授

高橋　哲也　　　　　順天堂大学保健医療学部理学療法学科　教授

池田　恵　　　　　　順天堂大学医療看護学部成人看護学　先任准教授

ナレーター

小島　エリ子　　　　NHK ワールドJAPAN TV/ラジオ　ナレーター

Marcellus Nealy　　順天堂大学医学部一般教育　准教授

Tom Kain　　　　　文京学院大学　非常勤講師

✚ 序文 ✚
Foreword

　心臓カテーテル検査で冠状動脈造影をする場合，撮像時に深呼吸をして息を止めてもらう．横隔膜を下げて，血管造影のコントラストをつけるためである．実際には「大きく息を吸ってー，はい，そこで止めてください」と声をかけ，そこで撮影を始める．5〜6秒で1回の撮像を終えると，「はい，楽にしてください」と言って次の造影検査に移る．

　私が研修医のときのことである．心臓カテーテル検査目的で入院してきた外国人の患者さんを担当した．病室で検査の目的や内容を英語で説明して，いざカテーテル検査室で検査を始めるときに，「あれ，呼吸の指示はなんと言うのだろう」と思っていると，指導医の先生が「Take a deep breath, please, and hold it!　………OK, breathe normally」と言って検査を進めた．

　最近，外国からの患者さんが受診される機会が増えているが，実際の臨床現場では専門医学的な説明よりも，かえって病棟や外来で話す日常会話で「あれっ」と思うことが多い．

　本書は医療関連職を目指す学生の基礎英語力を向上させると共に，臨床現場で患者さんと多職種の医療者で交わされる必要なコミュニケーション技術を習得して，国際的医療人を目指せるよう企画編集されている．

　自己紹介から始まり，患者さんとそのご家族とどのように話していくか，検査や治療の基本的な説明，栄養状態や生活スタイルの把握，そして高齢者医療，医療の多様性，最後に災害医療とチーム医療の項目別に主に Listening, Vocabulary, Grammar, Reading, Speaking & writing そして Language corner で構成され，医療現場で使える英語が知らず知らずのうちに身につくと共に，国際的なセンスが磨かれる．医療の専門家を目指す学生だけではなく，医療現場で働いている専門家の皆さんにも是非使って，楽しんで学んでもらいたい．

2022 年 2 月

監修者　代田 浩之

目次
Contents

✚ 本書の使い方 ✚
How to use the book

This textbook will allow you to help your students improve their language ability and help deepen their understanding of issues related to international health care. In this way, you can help your students become more well-rounded healthcare professionals. The topics are not difficult to understand. They do not require any special medical knowledge. Learners need only an openness to learning new ideas and a willingness to embrace the philosophical side of health care.

By the end of this course, students should have a better awareness of how to use active listening, speak with empathy, deliver bad news to their patients, talk to patients and their families, and other skills that are crucial to healthcare. One of the best things about this textbook is that students can use the information presented in each chapter in their daily practice. It doesn't matter what language they speak. For example, communicating with patients in a way that shows respect and empathy is a universal concept that goes beyond language. Not only will your students be able to improve their listening, grammar, and vocabulary, but they will also be able to improve their understanding of general healthcare. To maximize the effectiveness of this text, we encourage all teachers to read up on the various topics discussed in each chapter.

以下のQRコードから南江堂ホームページ上にある音声データ一覧に直接アクセスできます．
音声は Listening practice **1, 2** に対応しています．

https://www.nankodo.co.jp/video/9784524228133/index.html

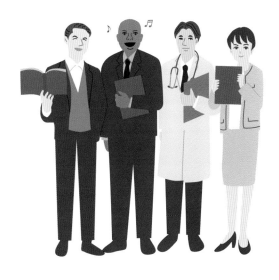

Chapter 1

Self-introductions

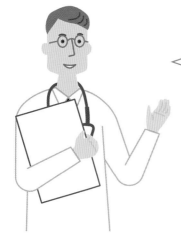

My name is Dr. Tanaka. I work at Nankodo Hospital.

Visiting the hospital or clinic can make some patients feel nervous. A warm, friendly greeting can help them relax. Self-introductions help you connect with patients. They help healthcare professionals establish rapport. When you speak to patients and their families, smile and introduce yourself. You should also appear confident and professional. Doing this right away will help patients immediately understand who you are and what to expect from you.

Listening practice 1

Read along while listening to the following conversation between a nurse and a patient.

◀ᵈ⁾ Track 1-1

Nurse: Hi, my name is Eriko. I am a nurse here at Nankodo Hospital. Can you tell me your name and date of birth, please?

Patient: Nice to meet you, Eriko. I am Naito. My birthday is February 25th, 1987.

Nurse: Nice to meet you, too, Mr. Naito. Can you tell me your full name, please?

Patient: Ryosuke Naito.

Nurse: Thank you, Mr. Naito.

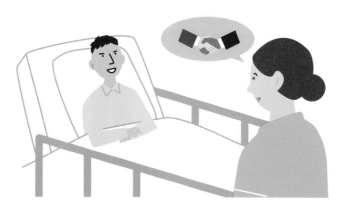

Listening practice 2

Listen to the following conversations. Write the missing words and phrases.

🔊 Track **1-2**

HCP: Hello. _____ _____ is Watanabe. I will be your _____ _____ today.

Patient: Hello, _____ Watanabe. It's lovely to _____ _____.

HCP: Can you _____ _____ your name, please?

Patient: Oh, sorry, someone called me in here, so I _____ you already knew my name.

HCP: Sorry about the _____. I do have a name here on the _____. I just need to double check to make sure you are the right _____.

Patient: No problem. I _____. You wouldn't want to work on the _____ person.

HCP: We sure _____!

Patient: My name is David.

HCP: Thanks, David. Just to be sure, may I have your _____ _____ as well, please?

Patient: Oh, right! My _____ name is David Anderson.

HCP: Thank you, David. It's _____ ____ _____ _____.

🔊 Track **1-3**

Nurse: Good afternoon. My name is Susan Allen. I am the _____ nurse for this Department.

Patient: It's nice to meet you, _____ _____.

Nurse: Please _____ _____ Susan.

Patient: It's nice to meet you, _____.

Nurse: It's nice to meet you, too. I have your name here on my chart, but _____ ____ ___ _____ I don't have the _____ _____, can you tell me your full name, please?

Patient: _____! My name is James Ranger.

Nurse: Thank you very much, _____ _____.

Patient: You're welcome, Susan. You _____ _____ _____ James.

Nurse: All right. Please _____ _____, James.

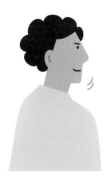
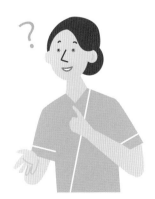

Vocabulary

Below is a list of key vocabulary for this chapter. Translate each word or phrase into your native language.

1. full name _____
2. first name _____
3. last name _____
4. rapport _____
5. comfortable _____
6. nervous _____
7. concern 名 _____
8. X-ray _____
9. CT _____
10. MRI _____
11. eye contact _____
12. confirm _____
13. confidence _____
14. behavior _____
15. assess _____
16. professionalism _____
17. mood _____
18. influence _____
19. impression _____
20. greet _____

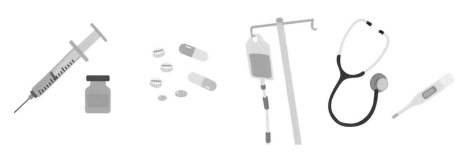

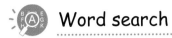 Word search

Find the words that are written in the list below. Words can be across, up and down, or diagonal.

```
H  V  Y  X  G  D  G  J  D  O  M  C  F  U  L  L  N  A  M  E
M  O  M  N  W  P  W  N  C  C  C  J  X  T  X  Z  X  D  P  C
B  M  U  G  Z  R  C  R  F  F  O  I  W  M  I  Y  F  E  F  N
F  V  M  H  I  M  Z  T  B  M  N  N  J  W  B  O  P  D  I  Z
X  I  L  R  P  C  D  U  G  P  F  F  Y  N  O  D  F  D  D  C
O  C  M  N  I  O  Z  X  Q  R  I  L  G  E  X  X  Z  D  E  Q
A  E  B  P  H  N  Z  L  P  O  R  U  N  R  Y  V  P  O  B  P
Y  M  L  F  R  C  U  S  Y  F  M  E  B  V  B  Z  J  V  T  X
F  O  V  K  A  E  W  F  D  E  T  N  C  O  S  I  O  X  Z  U
F  O  V  X  N  R  S  W  Y  S  X  C  N  U  H  X  C  N  J  J
Q  D  S  P  C  N  V  S  X  S  R  E  W  S  J  Q  C  F  S  U
J  J  Y  H  N  E  B  O  I  I  Y  G  W  N  B  M  O  R  D  N
Y  N  N  J  L  C  C  A  U  O  J  R  A  Z  E  H  N  G  N  G
S  W  X  L  F  N  B  L  B  N  N  A  I  I  H  G  F  G  L  Z
B  X  K  X  W  D  E  A  C  A  T  P  R  V  A  G  I  R  K  G
C  O  M  F  O  R  T  A  B  L  E  P  N  J  V  I  D  E  M  C
L  G  S  L  M  O  E  O  N  I  L  O  I  O  I  G  E  E  O  F
Q  Z  V  J  R  L  S  Q  J  S  X  R  S  Q  O  V  N  T  Z  C
U  U  A  B  I  B  E  V  T  M  Y  T  J  X  R  K  C  E  T  X
A  S  S  E  S  S  Y  C  J  O  Q  J  B  H  B  D  E  R  J  A
```

FULL NAME	RAPPORT	COMFORTABLE	NERVOUS
CONCERN	CT	MRI	CONFIRM
CONFIDENCE	BEHAVIOR	ASSESS	PROFESSIONALISM
MOOD	INFLUENCE	IMPRESSION	GREET

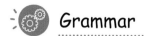 **Grammar**

Present tense (simple present)

The simple present tense is used in a variety of situations. Here are some common uses.

▶ **To show repeated actions or habits, unchanging situations, or general truths**

Ex I **work** at Nankodo Hospital. (repeated action/habit)

Ex My name **is** Dr. Tanaka. (unchanging situation)

Ex A smile **gives** people a good impression. (general truth)

▶ **To show fixed situations or routines**

Ex The hospital **opens** at 9 AM.

Ex Dinner **starts** at 7 PM sharp.

Ex I usually **wake up** at 6 AM.

▶ **To show the timing of a future action with words like** *after, when, before, as soon as,* **and** *until*

Ex I will call you when I **finish** the operation. (*not* "when I will finish")

Ex Try not to be nervous when you **introduce** yourself. (*not* "when you will introduce")

Ex Before you **go** home, please take a pamphlet. (*not* "before you will go")

Fill in the blanks below with the appropriate verb from the list below. Use the simple present tense and remember to match the verb to the subject.

Ex "He goes," *not* "He go".

> clean / go / be / pull / work

1. Hello. My name _____ Mari.

2. The patient will need to check her blood pressure before she _____ to the examination room.

3. Gravity _____ my feet to the ground.

4. She always _____ her house on Sunday mornings.

5. Doctors, nurses, radiologists, and pharmacists all _____ very hard.

Past tense (simple past)

The simple past tense is used for things that happened before now.

▶ **To describe a completed action in a time before now**

Ex She **went** to the hospital yesterday.

Ex I **graduated** from medical school 10 years ago.

Ex The patient **asked** for some advice.

▶ **The past tense is also used to describe more than one past occurrence in the same sentence**

Ex The patient **sat down** and **explained** her symptoms.

Ex Dr. Suzuki **gave** the patient a prescription and **told** him to get some rest.

Ex She **picked up** her mobile phone and **sent** a message.

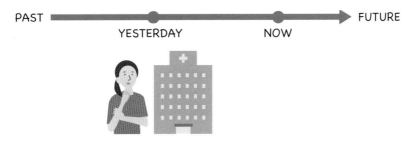

Fill in the blanks below with the appropriate verb from the list below. Use the simple past tense.

> receive / see / start / finish / be

1. The doctor _____ a letter from a patient the week before last.

2. Mary _____ him at the hospital yesterday.

3. The renovation of this building _____ in 1990.

4. He _____ assessing the patient and sent her home.

5. The coffee shop _____ full of young people last week.

Reading

Read the following passage. Answer the questions in the box below.

What patients think about you when they first meet you is important. In a few short minutes or seconds, they will decide if they can trust you. They will also decide if you are the person they can speak to openly. They will check your professionalism and sincerity. Whatever they decide will greatly influence their behavior toward you as a healthcare professional. That is why it is important to introduce yourself well.

There are several things you must keep in mind when introducing yourself. You should speak clearly and with confidence. Even if you are a shy person, you must appear confident in front of patients and their families. Be sure to get your patient's full name, even if it is written on a chart. This will not only help to confirm that you have the right person, but also help to establish a personal connection. You should be careful to match the patients' moods. If they are in deep pain, for example, a smile might make them feel as if you are not taking their condition seriously. You should also be aware of your vocal tone and speed. Your voice should show compassion, and you should talk at a speed that is understandable but not condescending.

When talking to patients, you should have good eye contact. Do not stare at your computer screen or your notes. Look directly at the patient. If the patient comes with a family member or friend, you must always speak directly to the patient when talking about his or her health and not to the person they brought to the hospital. For example, if the patient uses a translator to ask questions, you should look at the patient when you give your answer not at the translator. Talking to a translator or family member instead of the patient directly could make the patient feel invisible and alone. On the other hand, directly talking to the patient shows that you have made him or her your priority. This will help you to establish a good trusting relationship.

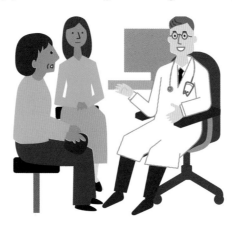

1. Why is your self-introduction important?
2. Why is showing confidence important?
3. Why shouldn't you smile or laugh when the patient is in deep pain?
4. Why should you always speak directly to the patient?
5. What are your overall thoughts about the reading?

Speaking & writing

1 Introduce yourself using the following sample phrases.

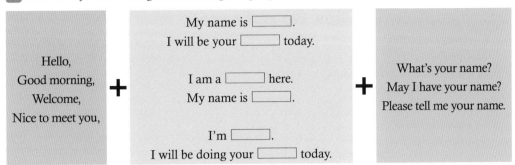

Hello,
Good morning,
Welcome,
Nice to meet you,

+

My name is ☐.
I will be your ☐ today.

I am a ☐ here.
My name is ☐.

I'm ☐.
I will be doing your ☐ today.

+

What's your name?
May I have your name?
Please tell me your name.

2 Combine the phrases in the orange, yellow, and green boxes to make three different introductions.

 ## What do you think?

Look at the following questions. Write down your opinion in response to each question. Share your opinions with the class, in small groups, or with your teacher.

1. Why are self-introductions important in your daily life?

2. Why are self-introductions important in the clinical setting?

3. In your culture, what are some things to consider when introducing yourself?

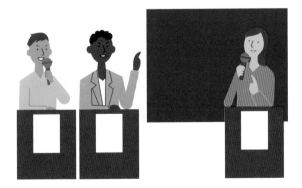

Language corner

Remember these important points when communicating in the clinical setting.

✓ Communication tips (to patients)

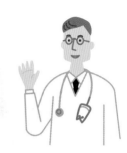

· Make eye contact
· Say hello
· Shake hands (if appropriate)
· Say your title
· Say your first and last name
· Say your function
· Ask for the patient's name
· Use Mr. or Ms. and their last name

> **Useful phrases**
>
> **Doctor** : Hello, my name is Dr. Allen. I am a radiologist at Nankodo. I will be doing your CT today. Can you tell me your name, please?
> **Patient**: My name is Lisa Watanabe.
> **Doctor** : Nice to meet you, Ms. Watanabe.

✓ Communication tips (to family)

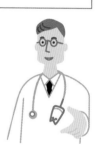

· First, Introduce yourself to the patient
· Second, Introduce yourself to the family
· Shake hands (if appropriate)
· Ask for the family members' names
· Confirm the relationship to the patient
· Look directly at the patient when talking about his or her health

> **Useful phrases**
>
> **Doctor** : Hello, my name is Dr. Naito. I am a kidney specialist. I will be doing your examination today. Can you tell me your name, please?
> **Patient**: My name is Lisa Watanabe.
> **Doctor** : Nice to meet you, Ms. Watanabe. (turn to the family) And you are...?
> **Family** : Mari Watanabe, I'm Lisa's sister.
> **Doctor** : It's a pleasure to meet you. (turn to the patient and continue)

✓ Communication tips (to coworkers)

· Say WHO you are
· Say WHAT you do
· Say WHERE you are from
· Say WHY you are there

> **Useful phrases**
>
> **Nurse** : Hi, I am Nurse, Stone. I work in the emergency room. I am taking care of Ms. Ida. I am here to get her chest X-rays.
> **Doctor** : Hello, Nurse Stone. I am Dr. Allen. I am the head radiologist here today. Please wait a moment. I will get the X-rays for you.
> **Nurse** : Thank you, Dr. Allen.

Professional profiles

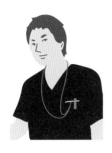

Name Kingo Hirasawa

Introduction Dr. Kingo Hirasawa is an endoscopic surgeon and associate professor who trains medical students and graduate students.

Comment My specialty is endoscopic surgery. I handle mild cases and also very severe cases. At the teaching hospital where I work, I'm responsible for training young doctors in the art of endoscopic surgery. I have done lots of research on the subject and written many papers. Throughout my career, I realized how important it is to learn English. I use it often in my work for research and connecting to the world. Without English, it is difficult for me to get the latest information on medical breakthroughs. Because English is the common language of healthcare, it is also difficult to share new discoveries with people in other countries if we cannot communicate in English. Sometimes we also have to care for patients who do not speak Japanese. Being able to speak even a little English helps those patients to feel at ease. For me, learning English is fun. I can meet many people from different countries. You don't have to be perfect. You just have to be sincere. A good relationship with your patients can start with a simple hello.

 Homework

Interview five of your classmates and collect the following information:

1. First name
2. Nationality and hometown
3. Three things the person likes
4. Three things the person doesn't like
5. The person's future dreams

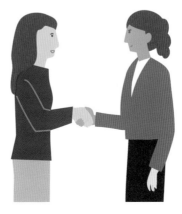

Chapter 2

Communicating with patients

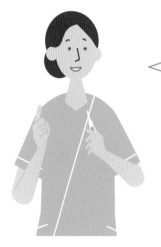

> I am a nurse in the dermatology department.

Getting patients to relax and share their feelings is the first step in the diagnostic process. When healthcare providers communicate with patients, they have to be active listeners. Active listening is a technique in which you use verbal and nonverbal cues to show patients that you are listening, acknowledge their emotions, and empathize with their concerns. When you communicate, using active listening will help your patients feel comfortable enough to share information and their emotions. Active listening helps you build trust and understanding between you and your patients.

Listening practice 1

Listen to the following lecture. Answer the following questions.

🔊 Track 2-1

1. Where does the word "rounds" originally come from?

2. Did the doctors and patients live in the same building?

3. What is the purpose of doing rounds? Explain two purposes.

4. What do you think about the system of doing rounds?

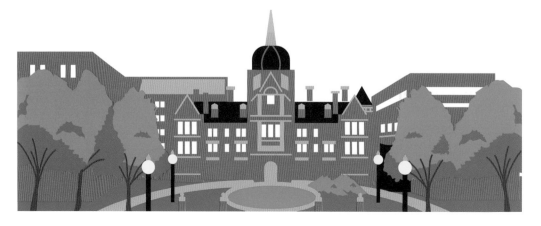

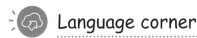 # Language corner

Remember these important active listening skills when communicating in the clinical setting.

✔ Use verbal cues

Verbal cues are words, phrases, or sentences that show you are listening to your patients.

Ex *reflecting, giving feedback, summarizing, minimal encouragers*

Useful phrases	
Reflecting	: "I don't feel well, and I have a headache." "I see you have a headache and don't feel so good. Let's see if we can find the cause."
Giving Feedback	: "I want you to take a moment to think. Is there anything you could have said or done differently?" (This is a way to gently correct patients when their words or actions are incorrect.)
Summarizing	: "Let me summarize what you have said to make sure I haven't missed anything."
Minimal Encouragers: Uh huh., I see., OK., Wow! , Really?	

✔ Use emotional labeling

Emotional labeling means recognizing your patients' emotions and saying them out loud.

Useful phrases
·I understand your feelings.
·You seem nervous about the test results.

✔ Do not use communication blockers

Communication blockers can prevent smooth conversation or make patients feel uncomfortable.

Ex *"why" questions, quick reassurance, preaching, digging into personal matters, interrupting*

Useful phrases
·Why did you do that?
·I can't believe you drink that much. Don't you know that drinking is bad for you?

✔ Use nonverbal cues

To know about the nonverbal cues, it is very helpful to understand the patients' feelings that are hard to express words.

Ex *posture, eye contact, facial expression, nodding, touch, hand gestures*

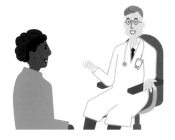

Vocabulary

Below is a list of key vocabulary for this chapter. Translate each word or phrase into your native language.

1. active listening _____

2. backchannel _____

3. informed consent _____

4. nonverbal communication _____

5. trust _____

6. posture _____

7. mirroring _____

8. refrain from _____

9. distraction _____

10. plain _____

11. empathy _____

12. questioning _____

13. reflection _____

14. open question _____

15. clarification _____

16. summarization _____

17. agree with _____

18. restating _____

19. sincerity _____

20. conclusion _____

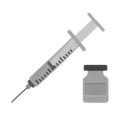

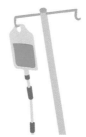
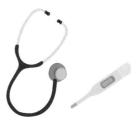

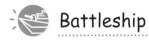 # Battleship

1. You have four ships of varying lengths. Place your ships on the map. Ships can be placed vertically and horizontally.
2. Take turns trying to find your partner's ships by stating coordinates, one from the left and one from the top (**Ex** Active/Empathy). When saying the coordinates, be sure to read the words out loud.
3. For example, if your submarine is at 10-A (Plain/Empathy) and 10-B (Plain/Questioning), and your partner calls out, "Is there something at Plain and Empathy? ", your partner will get a point because he or she will have found part of your ship.
4. The winner is the one who finds all of his or her partner's ships first or has the most points.

| Battleship | | | | | | Cruiser | | | |
| Carrier | | | | | | Submarine | | | |

My Ships		A Empathy	B Questioning	C Reflection	D Open question	E Clarification	F Summarization	G Agree with	H Restating	I Sincerity	J Conclusion
1	Active										
2	Backchannel										
3	Consent										
4	Nonverbal										
5	Trust										
6	Posture										
7	Mirroring										
8	Refrain from										
9	Distraction										
10	Plain										

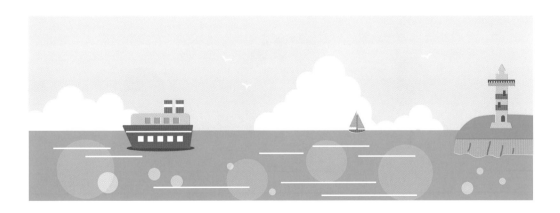

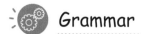 **Grammar**

Nouns

▶ **Nouns are names of people, places, and things**

`Ex` *dog, apple, information, the United States, woman*

▶ **English has countable nouns and uncountable nouns**

`Ex` Countable nouns: pen/pens, book/books

`Ex` Uncountable nouns: knowledge, furniture

▶ **Gender-neutral nouns are preferable when possible**

`Ex` △ businessman/○ businessperson

Articles

Articles are used before nouns. Words like *the, a,* and *an* are articles. There are two types of articles in English: indefinite and definite.

▶ **Indefinite articles**

"A" and "an" are indefinite articles. They are used when we mention something for the first time or to indicate something is one of many.

`Ex` I want **a** new watch. (*not* "I want new watch")

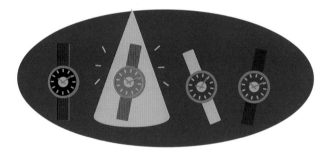

▶ **Definite article**

"The" is a definite article. We use "the" whenever the noun has been previously introduced or is clear in the mind of the speaker and the listener.

`Ex` **The** patient needs close monitoring.

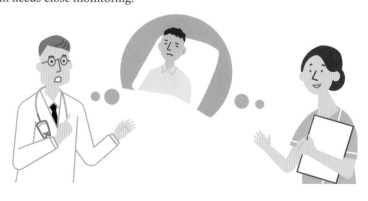

Possessives

Possessive adjectives show what or whom something belongs to.

▸ Possessive adjectives for regular nouns

Possessive adjectives for regular nouns show possession. In most cases, you form the possessive by adding an apostrophe and "s" to the noun (-'s). To make a possessive of a plural noun ending in "s," you just add an apostrophe at the end (-s').

Ex A doctor**'s** job is to improve patients**'** health. (*not* "patients's")

▸ Possessive adjectives for pronouns

Possessive adjectives for pronouns are, for example, *my*, *your*, *his*, *her*, *its*, and *their*. These are used to show that the pronoun they determine has possession of a noun.

Ex Could I see **his** chart?

▸ Possessive pronouns

Possessive pronouns include *mine*, *yours*, *his*, *hers*, and *theirs*. These can replace possessive nouns as either the subject or the object of a clause.

Ex This is your list of patients. Where's **mine**? (= **my** list)

---

1 Fill in the blanks with the missing words. Choose either "the" or "a."

1. I want to see _____ doctor who specializes in diabetes.

2. _____ moon is really beautiful tonight.

3. Who is _____ man standing next to Nurse Saito?

2 Circle the wrong word and write the correct answer. Pay attention to the possessive forms.

1. The doctor agreed with the nurses's recommendation.   (   )

2. Ms. Uchida has some questions about she's medication.   (   )

3. Let me ask you some questions about the symptoms of you.   (   )

Reading

Read the following passage. Answer the questions in the box below.

Being an active listener makes it more effective to communicate with patients and their families. It also helps them to have trust in your ability to perform medical examinations. Under the heading of active listening, there are many techniques that can be used. One of those is backchanneling.

Backchanneling is a way of providing signals to the speaker that you are listening to what they are saying. There are verbal and nonverbal backchannels. Verbal backchannels can be vocal sounds or short phrases like *Uh huh.*, *I see.*, *Right.*, and so on. Nonverbal backchannels are usually done with a head nod.

Backchanneling can also be used to give listener feedback. For example, it can be used to show approval ("I know, right?"). It can be used to reflect a question back to the listener (Speaker: "What do you think I did then?" Listener: "What did you do?"). Backchanneling can also be used to show emotions such as being surprised ("Wow!"), disappointed ("Oh no."), uncertain ("I don't know about that."), or sarcastic ("Oh, is that so?").

There are some cultural and linguistic differences. Japanese speakers, for example, use backchanneling much more than other language speakers. Usage of backchannels in Japanese is about three times more than in American English. The habit of using backchannels in Japanese conversation can be transferred to other languages. When native Japanese speakers communicate in English, they tend to use about twice as many backchannels as Americans. Sometimes, people who come from countries where backchanneling is used less, the increased amount of backchanneling from Japanese speakers can seem like too much and make the Japanese healthcare professionals seem insincere. Backchanneling should always be used with just the right amount of balance.

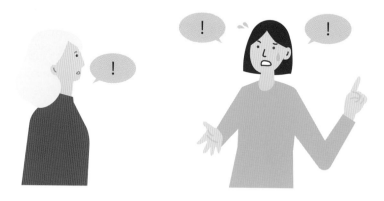

1. Can you think of sounds, words, phrases, or gestures that can be used for backchanneling in your native language? Please make a list and describe how they can be used. (Ex to show agreement, disappointment, etc.)
2. Why is too much backchanneling bad ?
3. If someone were to ask you to describe backchanneling, what would you say?

🖊 Speaking & writing

Match each illustration with the active listening skills you learned in this chapter.

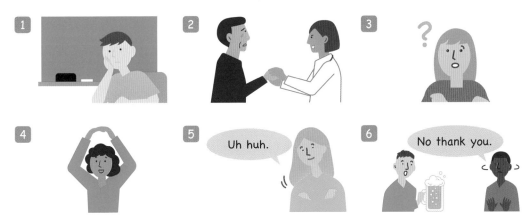

empathy / questioning / summarization / distraction / refrain from
backchannel / nonverbal communication / clarification

	Words / Phrases		Words / Phrases
1.		**4.**	
2.		**5.**	
3.		**6.**	

💬 What do you think?

Look at the following questions. Write down your opinion in response to each question. Share your opinions with the class, in small groups, or with your teacher.

1. What kind of behaviors do you think would block communication with people?

2. Why do "Why" questions make some patients feel defensive?

3. What kind of nonverbal communication skills can you come up with, and in what situations do you think they are effective to use?

Listening practice 2

Listen to the following conversation between a professor and a student. Write the missing words and phrases.

🔊 Track 2-2

Professor: Today, I'll explain _____ _____ you should keep in mind while interacting with patients. First, all healthcare professionals should learn _____ _____.

Student: What is that?

Professor: Active listening is a _____ style that focuses on the importance of _____ first. The goal is to listen to the patient as _____ as possible.

Student: Can you give me an _____?

Professor: Well, doctors should _____ emotions by saying out loud the _____ they think the patient might be experiencing. If a patient seems afraid, the doctor might say, "I can _____ that you're afraid." This will be a sign that the doctor is _____ _____ to his or her patient.

Student: I see. So active listening is about showing you are _____ paying attention.

Professor: That's correct.

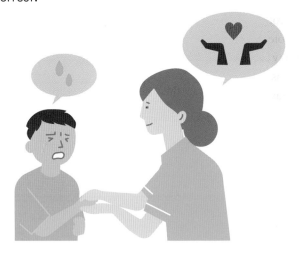

💡 Key Points

Active listening helps to build a relationship between healthcare providers and their patients. When patients feel their healthcare providers are sincerely listening to them, they can better trust their healthcare providers' judgment. Research has shown that active listening leads to better clinical outcomes. That's because when patients trust their healthcare providers, they are more willing to follow treatment plans and advice on how to stay healthy. Active listening is all about recognizing the emotions of patients and showing empathy. When learning to communicate with patients, it is a great idea to start with active listening.

Early X-ray equipment

Read the following passage. Answer the questions written in the box below.

X-rays are now essential devices in medical examinations. The word X-ray is used in English. In Japanese, it's called Roentgen and was named after the person who discovered X-ray radiation.

The German physicist Wilhelm Conrad Röntgen discovered radiation in December 1895. The news quickly spread around the world. Four scholars quickly succeeded in doing X-ray photography in Japan the following year. After that, physicians began to use X-ray images of bones to diagnose bone fractures and to identify the presence of foreign bodies. However, it was not until the Taisho era (1912–1926) that X-rays came to be widely used as medical diagnostic equipment. Juntendo Hospital, Department of Radiology was one of the earliest clinics to use X-rays. They invited Goichi Fujinami, a radiologist who had just returned from studying in Germany, to do the procedure.

Photo (1) shows the examination room where X-rays were done in 1919. The examiner's protective equipment seems rather bulky. However, at that time, they needed to protect themselves in this way since much was still unknown about the nature of X-ray radiation. Photo (2) shows the first X-ray device at Juntendo Hospital in 1919. It was a DC-sensing coil device called "Avex." Equipped in 2nd Internal Medicine X-ray room 1933.

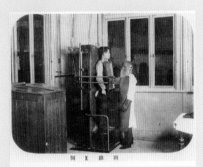 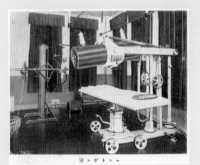

Photo (1)
[Reproduced with permission and copyright of Juntendo University website]

Photo (2)
[Reproduced with permission and copyright of Juntendo University website]

1. Who invented the X-ray?
2. When did X-ray examinations begin at Juntendo Hospital?
3. Why did they need extreme protection when using the X-ray machine?
4. Who performed the first X-ray at Juntendo Hospital?
5. What kind of medical equipment do you think will be developed in the future?

Chapter 3

Communicating with family

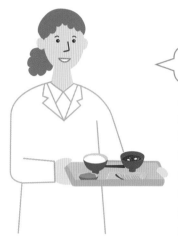

> Your mother looks better than yesterday.

A trust-based relationship with patients and their families is essential for treatment and meeting mutual expectations. This is true not only for doctors but also for any medical staff that work with patients and their families. It is essential to recognize family members as a source of valuable information and support. Family members can advocate, express concerns, make decisions, remember doctors' instructions, observe, and interpret on behalf of the patient.

Listening practice 1

Listen to the following sentences. Which word or phrase best matches the sentence you hear?

 Track 3-1

> active listening / informed consent / trust /posture /
> mirroring / distraction / open question / clarification /
> summarization / empathy

	Words / Phrases		Words / Phrases
1.		6.	
2.		7.	
3.		8.	
4.		9.	
5.		10.	

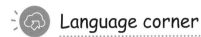

Language corner

Remember these important active listening skills when communicating in the clinical setting.

✔ Use verbal cues

Verbal cues are words, phrases, or sentences that show you are listening to your patients. Below are some more types of verbal cues.

Ex *"I" messages, redirecting, consequences, validation*

✔ "I" messages

These are statements about your own feelings, ideas, and beliefs. They should be said in a way that does not sound arrogant.

> Useful phrases
> ·I understand your situation and will do my best to help you.

✔ Redirecting

This is a way to change the subject or get the conversation back on subject.

> Useful phrases
> ·Thank you for that story about your neighbor. Now, let's talk more about your health.

✔ Consequences

This is a way of gently getting patients to think about the result of their actions.

> Useful phrases
> ·Have you thought about how bad your symptoms will be if you stop taking the medications?

✔ Validation

This is a way of letting patients know it is OK to feel what they are feeling, so they can feel more comfortable.

> Useful phrases
> ·What you are feeling is perfectly normal.

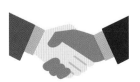 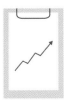 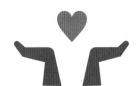

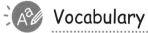 ## Vocabulary

Below is a list of key vocabulary for this chapter. Translate each word or phrase into your native language.

1. appointment _____

2. observer _____

3. confidential information _____

4. decision-making _____

5. interpretation _____

6. relative _____

7. impair _____

8. ward _____

9. visual aid _____

10. explaining _____

11. word choice _____

12. essential _____

13. reassurance _____

14. turn-taking _____

15. validation _____

16. effective pause _____

17. "I" message _____

18. redirecting _____

19. consequence _____

20. emergency contact _____

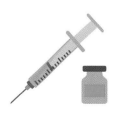 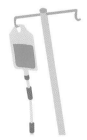 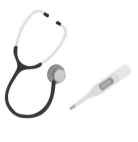

Word maze

Help the patient find the radiology department. Start from the center of the maze. Read the clues written below to find the correct path to the radiology department. Each word must be connected to the next word by a straight line. Which room is it in? Follow the line to find the answer.

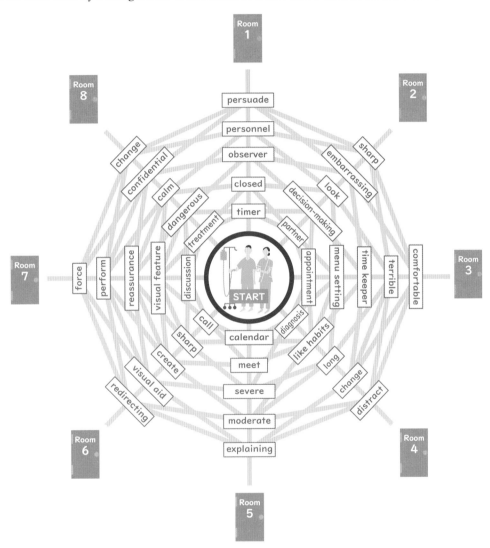

1. A word that means a set date and time.
2. A phrase that means making choices.
3. A word that means someone who watches.
4. A word that means something must be kept secret.
5. A word that describes the act of removing doubts and fears.
6. A thing we use to help explain what we mean.
7. An action we do to communicate information.
8. An action we do to change the conversation.

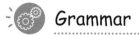 Grammar

Comparatives

In medical settings, people often compare two conditions, two medications, or two treatment options. Comparatives allow you to compare two things. Often, we use adjectives and adverbs to describe the differences between two things.

▶ **Adjectives**

Look at these two pieces of yarn. A and B have different lengths. If you want to explain that difference, you can use the adjectives "short" or "long" in the comparative. An adjective comparative describes differences in the way things are.

A **is** longer **than** B. **/** B **is** shorter **than** A.

The pattern is simple for adjectives:
A + "be" verb + comparative adjective **+ than + B.**

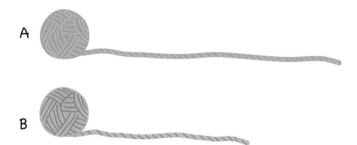

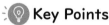 Key Points

- Most comparative adjectives are formed by adding "–er" to the end of the adjective.
  Ex long → longer / nice → nicer
- There are also some irregular comparatives.
  Ex good → better / bad → worse
- For most longer adjectives (with two or more syllables), you make the comparative by adding "more" or "less" in front of the adjective.
  Ex dangerous → less dangerous / helpful → more helpful

▸Adverbs

Imagine that Jim and Kevin both have colds. Jim recovered fully in three days, but Kevin took five days to recover. In this case, you could use a comparative adverb to show the difference between Jim and Kevin. A comparative adverb describes a difference in how someone does something (not how something is).

Jim **recovered** more quickly **than** Kevin. / Kevin **recovered** more slowly **than** Jim.

The pattern for comparative adverbs is:
A + regular verb + (object, etc.) + comparative adverb **+ than + B + (regular verb).**

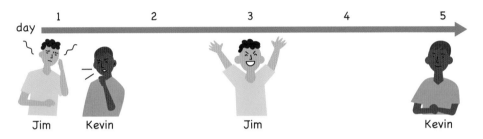

> ### 🔍 Key Points
>
> • The rules for forming comparative adverbs are basically the same as those for comparative adjectives.
>   Ex late → later / hard → harder / easily → more easily
> • Common irregular adverbs include "well," whose comparative form is "better."
>   Ex You look better than yesterday. (*not* "more well")

Make a sentence for each of the following situations. Use comparative adjectives or adverbs.

1. Dr. Ishikawa's age: 29 / Dr. Funakoshi's age: 37

2. Drug A's effectiveness rate: 85% / Drug B's effectiveness rate: 92%

3. Surgery A's cost: 300,000 yen / Surgery B's cost: 250,000 yen

4. Patient A visits the hospital twice a month / Patient B visits the hospital every week

5. The patient felt bad yesterday / The patient feels good today

Read the following passage. Answer the questions in the box below.

Communicating with the family is just as important as communicating directly with the patient. Often, family members contribute to important decision-making. They can also provide psychological and financial support. When patients cannot care for themselves, family members may also become the main caregiver. It is important to make sure your communication with the family is smooth so that you can create a good relationship. Active listening can certainly help with this. In active listening, healthcare providers show empathy, acknowledge emotions, and offer reassurance.

This can be done with a smile, good eye contact, good posture, and appropriate touching. Appropriate touching, such as putting your hand on a shoulder when someone is going through negative emotions, is common in many countries. However, you should observe the person closely to see if they are OK with being touched. If they are not, you should stop immediately.

There are other useful active listening skills, such as reflecting, which is briefly repeating back what the speaker has said to show you have understood. Reflecting is usually done midway through explanation. Another active listening skill is summarizing, which is done at the end by repeating everything important the person has said. Usually, you only summarize clinically relevant information or information that shows you understand the person's thoughts, concerns, and expectations. Validation is also useful. It is a statement you give to let someone know that it is OK to feel the way that they are feeling. Validation allows people to release the shame, guilt, or embarrassment they may have as a result of their emotional state. Phrases like "What you are feeling is understandable." help to validate the person's feelings.

Please remember that your focus should always be on the patient. If there are family members present, your eye contact and speech should always be directed towards the patient. If your patient cannot speak your language and is using a translator, you should look directly at the patient. If you don't do that, the patient may feel ignored and insignificant.

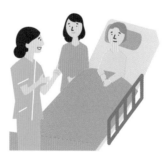

1. Why is it important to communicate properly with the patients' family members?
2. Why is eye contact important?
3. What are the active listening skills mentioned in the reading?
4. Of the skills you listed in question 3, which one is the most difficult to master and why ?
5. Describe a moment when you felt as if someone wasn't listening to you. How did you feel?

Speaking & writing

Write down all the types of emotion you can think of. If you don't know the words in English, check with your dictionary.

Ex *happy, angry, sad, relaxed*

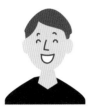 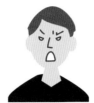 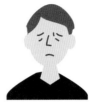 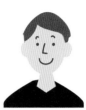

 ## What do you think?

Look at the following questions. Write down your opinion in response to each question. Share your opinions with the class, in small groups, or with your teacher.

1. What roles do patient's family members play in the patient's life?
2. When speaking with healthcare professionals, what sort of requests do you think family members might make?
3. How do healthcare professionals establish trust with patients and family members?
4. A father brings his 10-year-old daughter to the clinic. Who should healthcare workers pay the most attention to and why?

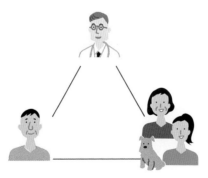

 Key Points

Dialogue with patients, family members and doctor is called the therapeutic triangle. The goal is to get information about patients' daily life, family relationships, and support systems. The therapeutic triangle helps improve medical care. When communicating with the family, always remember to keep patients at the center of attention. Even if the patient does not speak your language, do not ignore them by speaking only to their family members or interpreters.

Listening practice 2

Listen to the following conversation between a nurse and a healthcare professional (HCP). Write the missing words and phrases.

🔊 Track 3-2

Nurse: Today's patient will arrive with his _____.

HCP: Can you tell me more about him?

Nurse: He is an _____ _____ man who is _____ _____. One of his family members will take on the _____ of translator.

HCP: I see. We should probably be careful about the _____ _____ as well as the _____ ____ _____. Not only should we speak slowly, but we should also use _____ _____ to give him _____ to respond.

Nurse: Yes, that is an excellent idea.

HCP: Also, let's pay attention to his verbal and nonverbal cues. _____ of his emotions and concerns may help him _____ more relaxed.

Nurse: OK, He's a cheerful person, He _____ to talk.

HCP: OK, then we will _____ the topic if the discussion _____ _____ _____. Let's be sure to discuss _____ _____ if the patient is not following _____ _____ _____.

Also, we should talk about _____ _____ _____ in helping him stick to the plan.

Nurse: I will do that.

HCP: Oh! I almost forgot. We have to make sure his family provides _____ _____ information and make ____ _____ for the next visit.

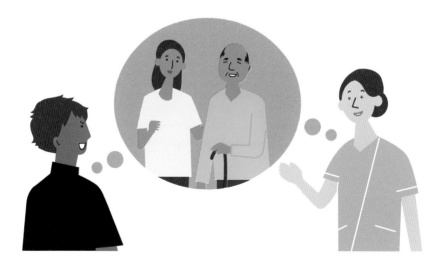

Medical interpreters

Medical interpreters are interpreters who help healthcare professionals and patients communicate when they speak a different language. Unlike common interpreters, they accompany patients through the whole process of their hospital visit. There are a wide range of situations where medical interpreters might be needed, from reception desks to pharmacies. Medical interpreters are sometimes needed during difficult situations such as emergencies, psychiatric care, and helping patients give informed consent. Volunteers, family and friends have often served as unofficial interpreters, but errors in translation sometimes leads to serious clinical consequences. To solve this problem, many institutions began training professional medical interpreters. At Juntendo University, Faculty of International Liberal Arts, students are able to acquire a wide range of knowledge about medical care and medical English, which is the basis for becoming a medical interpreter. Also, a new graduate course of medical interpreting was established at Juntendo University Graduate School of Medicine in 2021. In this way, Juntendo University is helping to bridge the gap between healthcare professionals and international patients.

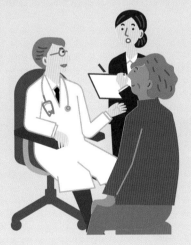

History taking

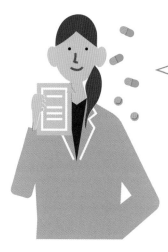

Do you take any medications?

When meeting a patient for the first time, a healthcare professional will take a medical history by asking questions. As you have learned in the previous two chapters, listening is very important, and careful listening can often result in a diagnosis. In many cases, physicians can make a diagnosis based solely on the patient's medical history. If the patient trusts you, they will usually speak more easily and openly, increasing the likelihood of you obtaining valuable medical information. Therefore, healthcare professionals should create an atmosphere that will make their patients feel comfortable and relaxed.

🎧 Listening practice 1

Listen to the following conversation between a medical social worker (MCW) and a patient. Write the missing words and phrases.

🔊 Track 4-1

MCW: Good morning. I'm a medical social worker, Henry Bracken. Please _____ ____ and _____ a seat.

Patient: Thank you.

MCW: I _____ _____ your chart and would like to confirm some details.

Patient: OK.

MCW: Your name is Alexis Tanaka, and _____ _____ ____ _____ is January 15th, _____, correct?

Patient: Yes.

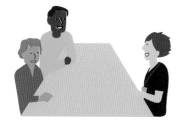

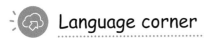

Language corner

Below are the basic steps of history taking and sample sentences you can use for each step.

✔ Step 1: Get the chief complaint

· How can I help you today?

✔ Step 2: Get the history of present illness using OPQRST

· Onset : "When did your symptoms start?"
· Palliation & provocation : "Is there anything that makes it better or worse?"
· Quality : "Can you describe the pain? Is it a dull pain, a sharp pain…"
· Region & radiation : "Which part of your stomach hurts? Is it the upper part, the middle…" "Do you feel pain anywhere else?" "Has the rash spread?"
· Severity & symptoms : "On a scale of 1 to 10, with 1 being very mild pain and 10 being a horrific pain, how bad is it?" "Have you noticed any other symptoms?"
· Timing : "Do the symptoms appear after you have done something or eaten something?" "Do the symptoms happen at certain times of the day?"

✔ Step 3: Get the medical history

· Have you had any other illnesses in the past?
· Are you taking any medications?

✔ Step 4: Get the family medical history

· Has anyone in your family had any serious illnesses?

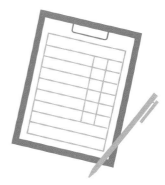

✔ Step 5: Get the social history

· Do you drink alcohol or smoke cigarettes?
· How much do you drink/smoke?
· What do you do for work?

✔ Step 6: Summarize

· I would like to summarize what we have talked about today.

✔ Step 7: Get the patient's thoughts (ICE)

· Ideas : What do you know about your condition?
· Concerns : Do you have any other concerns?
· Expectations : What do you expect moving forward?

※ Please note that history taking also requires a review of relevant systems, which has been omitted from this text.

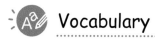 Vocabulary

Below is a list of key vocabulary for this chapter. Translate each word or phrase into your native language.

1. privacy _____

2. introduction _____

3. chief complaint _____

4. onset _____

5. palliation _____

6. quality _____

7. region _____

8. radiation _____

9. symptom _____

10. severity _____

11. time _____

12. emotional pain _____

13. physical pain _____

14. medical history _____

15. family history _____

16. social history _____

17. summary _____

18. idea _____

19. provocation _____

20. expectation _____

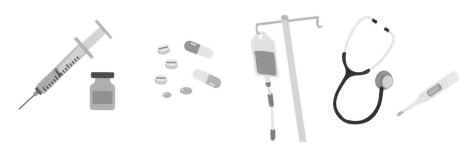

Crossword

Using the hints below, fill in the words to the puzzle.

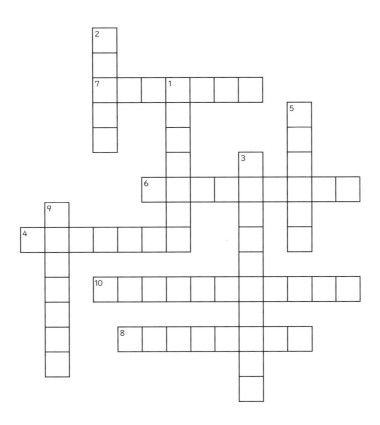

1. This is protected information about individuals and families.
2. This is when the symptoms began.
3. This is making the symptoms feel better.
4. This describes a distinguishing attribute.
5. This tells us where the patients are experiencing pain.
6. This is a word that describes the movement of pain.
7. This is a signal the body gives us to let us know when we are injured or ill.
8. This is how bad pain and other symptoms feel.
9. This is a review of everything you talked about with your patient.
10. This is something that makes a symptom worse.

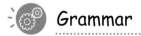 # Grammar

Interrogative

In English, there are many different types of sentences. The most common type is the declarative form. It gives information. Here are some examples of that basic form.

It is cold today.
I take medications.
I will have surgery tomorrow.
The nurse can answer your questions.
Reception hours **start** at 9 AM.

Those types of sentences *give* information. But what if you need to *get* information from someone? In that case, you need to ask a question. That's when you use the interrogative (question) form. Imagine that the five sentences above are the answers to five questions. Here's what the questions would look like.

Is it cold today?
Do you take any medications?
Will you have surgery tomorrow?
Can the nurse answer my questions?
When do reception hours **start**?

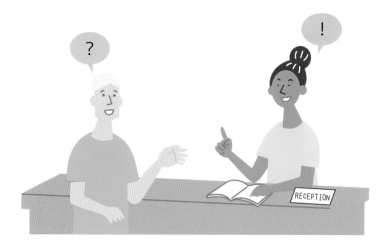

▶ Basic patterns for interrogative sentences

There are four basic patterns for interrogative sentences.

(1) Be verb + subject + other information
   Ex Are you all right?
(2) Auxiliary verb + subject + verb + other information
   Ex Does he want some water?
(3) Question word + be verb + subject + other information
   Ex How is your mother doing?
(4) Question word + auxiliary verb + subject + verb + other information
   Ex What should I write on this form?

💡 Key Points

When you make an interrogative sentence, just remember that it will always begin with either a be verb, an auxiliary verb (*do, can, should*, etc.), or a question word (*who, what, when, where, why,* or *how*).

Make an interrogative (question) sentence for each of the answers written below.

Ex Answer: I walked to work this morning. (Start with an auxiliary verb.)
   ➡ Interrogative sentence: Did you walk to work this morning?

1. Answer: I started having a headache last night. (Start with "When.")

2. Answer: I understood the instructions. (Start with an auxiliary verb.)

3. Answer: The symptoms were bad. (Start with a "be" verb.)

4. Answer: I take several medications. (Start with a question word.)

5. Answer: You can enter the examination room now. (Start with an auxiliary verb.)

Read the following passage. Answer the questions in the box below.

Medical history taking, when properly sequenced and carefully conducted, can often reveal an accurate diagnosis. Medical tests, while important, are often used to confirm a diagnosis that has been made during history taking. They should never substitute for talking with the patient and collecting diagnostically relevant information. Many healthcare professionals and healthcare researchers have agreed with this idea. Fortunately, healthcare students will soon have the opportunity to experience it themselves.

In order to take a patient history, it is important for healthcare professionals and patients to have clear communication. Mutual respect between the doctor and the patient is also important. All healthcare professionals have the best chance of experiencing positive patient attitudes when they use active listening. If patients feel they are being listened to, they are more likely to provide a complete and more accurate picture of their health condition. More detailed information means that healthcare professionals will be more likely to understand their patients' health problems and make good decisions.

During a normal day, healthcare professional face many problems and many distractions. For that reason, the average healthcare professionals is often very busy and has little time. Taking a thorough history requires healthcare professional to spend time with their patients. Some doctors, nurses, and other healthcare professionals may feel there's not enough time to take a history as they were taught to do in school. However, using a carefully crafted history-taking protocol, along with much practice, healthcare professionals can become good at quickly finding the cause of their patients' medical problems. Health issues often have a long history. The rewards of history-taking make it worth the effort for healthcare professionals and their patients.

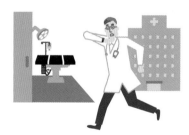

1. What is the purpose of doing a proper medical history?
2. What does a healthcare professional need to take a proper history?
3. Why do you think patients are more likely to share information if they feel you are listening to them?
4. Even when doctors and other healthcare professionals are busy, they must take time to listen to their patients. Please explain in your own words why this might be true.
5. What are your general thoughts about history–taking and communication with patients?

Speaking & writing

Imagine your future patients. What kind of people will they be? Please write two imaginary stories about a man and a woman who have gone to the hospital for a checkup. Describe their age, appearance, occupation, family life, personal life, and health situation.

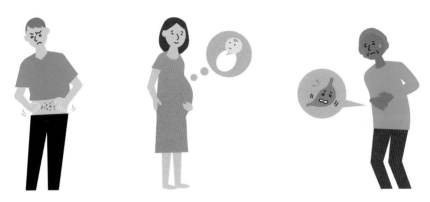

 ## What do you think?

Look at the following questions. Write down your opinion in response to each question. Share your opinions with the class, in small groups, or with your teacher.

1. What are some of the illnesses patients might not want to talk about with others?
2. Please explain why you chose the diseases you listed for question 1.
3. What are some things you can do to make it easier for the patient to talk about their illness?

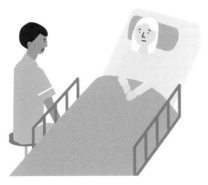

Listening practice 2

Listen to the following conversation between a doctor and a patient. Complete the notes below. If there is no corresponding answer, leave the answer space blank.

🔊 Track4-2

Chief complaint: _____

Onset: _____

Palliation & provocation: _____

Quality: _____

Region: _____

Radiation: _____

Severity: _____

Symptoms: _____

Timing: _____

🔊 Track4-3

Chief complaint: _____

Onset: _____

Palliation & provocation: _____

Quality: _____

Region: _____

Radiation: _____

Severity: _____

Symptoms: _____

Timing: _____

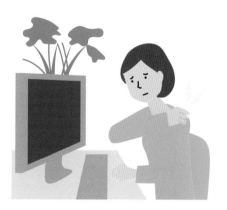 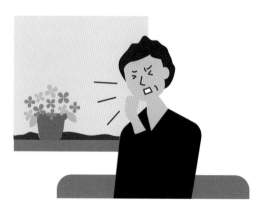

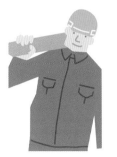

Name Daniel Washington

Patient info 55-year-old male, he came to the hospital because he had been experiencing discomfort and pain in his chest. Sometimes, he also found it difficult to breathe.

Comment Daniel is a construction worker. He is the father of three children. His son is 25 years old and lives in Tokyo. His twin daughters are 22 years old. For the past couple of years, Daniel has had high blood pressure. He is taking medication for it. Besides hypertension, he has not had any major health issues in the past. His wife is worried about him because his father and grandfather both died of a heart attack. She explained to the doctor that Daniel loves to eat meat, cheese, and other foods that are high in cholesterol. He also loves to drink alcohol. Daniel agreed with his wife and added that he didn't like the taste of vegetables. He thinks that eating them makes him feel like a rabbit. Daniel loves sports. His favorites are American football and baseball. Daniel and his wife were visiting their son in Tokyo when his symptoms first appeared.

 ## Homework

Work in pairs to practice history taking. One person will play the role of patient, and the other will play the role of doctor. Take turns getting a medical history from each other.

Ex **Doctor:** Hello, my name is Dr. Naito. May I have your name, please?
Patient: I'm Leslie Chan. Nice to meet you.

4

History taking

5 Basic instructions

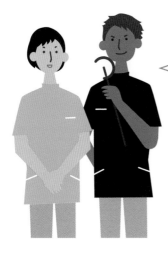

Hold your breath.

Having your body examined can be an uncomfortable experience. Knowing how to convey basic instructions in a polite and comprehensible manner is a vital skill in helping patients feel comfortable when getting X-rayed and undergoing tests and procedures. The words and phrases introduced in this chapter will ensure that you and your patients feel relaxed and confident.

Listening practice 1

Listen to the following conversation between a radiological technologist (RT) and a patient. Write the missing words and phrases.

🔊 **Track 5-1**

RT: Please come in. _____ ____ _____ name and birthday, please.

Patient: I'm Matthew Rodriguez. My birthday is February 28th, 1985.

RT: Thank you, Mr. Rodriguez. I'd like to take some X-rays of your chest now. Could you take off your shirt please and _____ ____ _____ ____ the white square, which is right next to you?

Patient: This one?

RT: Yes, that's the one. Could you _____ ___ _____ ____ ____ ____?

Patient: Here?

RT: That's perfect. Now please _____ _____ _____ _____ _____ _____ and hold them there.

Patient: Like this?

RT: Yes. Very good. Please _____ _____.

RT: Now, please _____ ___ _____ _____ and _____ ___.

RT: Very good. Now please _____ _____ .

Listening practice 2

Listen to the following conversation between a physical therapist (PT) and a patient. Write the missing words and phrases.

🔊 Track 5-2

PT: OK. Mrs. Johnson, can you _____ _____ for me, please? Slowly, slowly. That's very good. Now I'd like for you to _____ your right arm. Could you raise it ___ _____ _____, please?

Patient: Like this?

PT: _____. I need you to raise your hand _____ your head like you're a student asking a question in class.

Patient: I see. Do you mean _____ _____?

PT: Yes, that's _____. Now, I want you to _____ _____ arm straight and _____ _____ arm slowly down back ____ _____ _____.

Patient: Like this?

PT: Yes, that's very good. OK, let's do the same with the left arm. _____ your left arm, please.

Patient: OK.

PT: Now, just like you did with the right arm, I want you to _____ ____ _____ and lower it slowly.

Patient: I can do that.

PT: You sure did an _____ _____, Mrs. Johnson. Now could you go to the bed and ____ _____, please?

Patient: It's way over there. I may need _____.

PT: I'm right here if you need me.

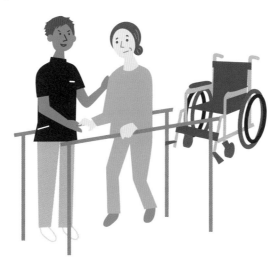

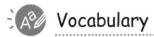 Vocabulary

Below is a list of key vocabulary for this chapter. Translate each word or phrase into your native language.

1. between

2. beside

3. in front of

4. to the right/left of

5. imperative

6. polite

7. calm

8. neutral

9. procedure

10. turn right/left

11. raise/lift

12. put

13. lower

14. turn

15. bend

16. straighten

17. breathe in/out

18. deep breath

19. hold your breath

20. lie down

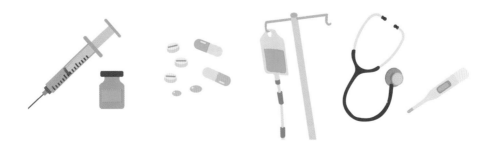

Match illustrations and words or phrases

Look at the illustrations below. Choose the word or phrase that matches the illustration. Also, write the part of the body that is depicted in the illustration.

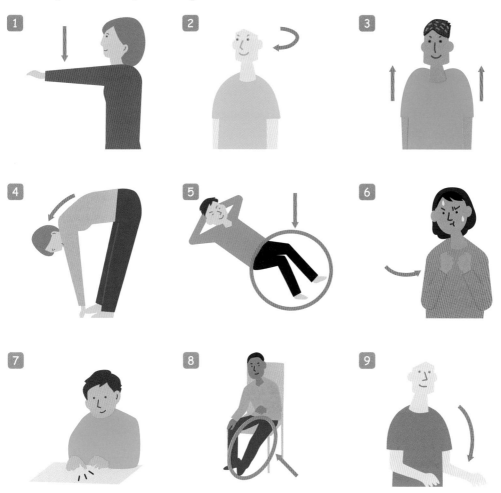

straighten / turn right / lie down / put / raise /
hold your breath / lower / in front of / bend

	Words / Phrases	Parts		Words / Phrases	Parts		Words / Phrases	Parts
1.			4.			7.		
2.			5.			8.		
3.			6.			9.		

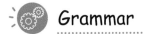 Grammar

Imperative

▸ **When you want to tell someone *to do* something (give an instruction)**

Imperatives are commands. These are useful when giving instructions to patients. To make an imperative sentence, use a "root" verb (a verb in its basic form) without including a subject.

Ex Hold your breath.

Ex Go down the hall and turn left.

▸ **When you want to tell someone *not to do* something**

When you want to tell someone not to do something, put "do not" in front of the root verb. You can also shorten "do not" to "don't."

Ex Do not lift your leg.

Ex Don't drive yourself home today.

▸ **When you want to give an instruction politely**

When giving instructions to patients, be sure to make your instructions polite.

There are many ways to make polite commands. Here are some examples. Of the four patterns below, patterns (3) and (4) are the politest.

(1) Please + imperative command.

   Ex Please turn your head to the left.

(2) Could you + imperative command?

   Ex Could you turn your head to the left?

(3) Could you + imperative command + , please?

   Ex Could you turn your head to the left, please?

(4) Could you + imperative command + for me, please?

   Ex Could you turn your head to the left for me, please?

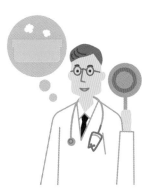 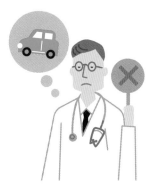

💡 Key Points

It's best to give polite instructions, but using the imperative form without "please" or "could you" isn't necessarily rude. Just make sure that you say the instruction in a courteous and friendly tone.

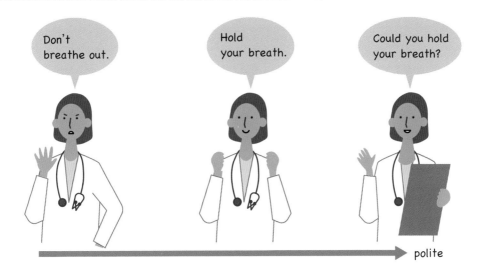

Don't breathe out.

Hold your breath.

Could you hold your breath?

polite

Using patterns 1–4 above, make polite requests for the following imperative sentences.

1. Roll up your sleeve.

2. Lie on your back.

3. Put this thermometer under your arm.

4. Take a deep breath.

5. Have a seat in the waiting room.

📖 Reading

Read the following passage. Answer the questions in the box below.

When you are giving instructions to patients, there are three key concepts to keep in mind.

First, be clear and concise. You can achieve this by communicating in simple and polite language. Using short sentences with simple language will help to make your message clear. You can reduce the stress that patients might feel by making your instructions less complicated and easy to follow. As instructional phrases are often repeated, memorizing these simple phrases will also make communication easier for both you and your patients.

Second, keeping your tone polite will put your patients at ease, and they will feel respected. Remember that it is not only what you say but how you say it that is important. Ask questions to make sure patients or their family members have understood your requests. For more complicated procedures, ask them to repeat the instructions back to you. If you communicate openly with your patients, they will feel comfortable enough to tell you if they have any questions or hesitation about your directions.

Finally, be pleasant and calm. When speaking with patients, it is best to use neutral and calm vocal tones. In general, people do not like to feel they are being commanded to do something. If patients feel something is being demanded or they have no personal choice, it might create a psychological barrier that makes the patient feel hesitant to do what you are asking. By using a neutral and calm voice, you can avoid this negativity and have a positive interaction with your patients.

Also, never forget that you must treat all patients equally regardless of their age, gender, nationality, or social status. All patients should be spoken to with the same level of respect and compassion. Because healthcare professionals are human, it is sometimes easy to forget this simple idea. It is important that you also observe your own habits when you interact with your patients. Giving instructions to patients is a large part of the work you will be doing. By remembering these key concepts, you can make that experience a pleasant one.

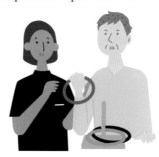

1. According to the passage, why should medical professionals give directions in short and simple sentences?
2. How can you create an open line of communication with your patients?
3. Why is it important to use a neutral and calm tone of voice?
4. What are the three key concepts mentioned in the passage?
5. Why is it bad to treat patients different based on age, gender, nationality, or social status?

Speaking & writing

Imagine you are a healthcare professional. Work in pairs. Take turns giving instructions to each other based on the following scenarios.

1. A radiological technologist giving a stomach exam
2. A physical therapist giving rehabilitation
3. A nurse giving a patient a shot

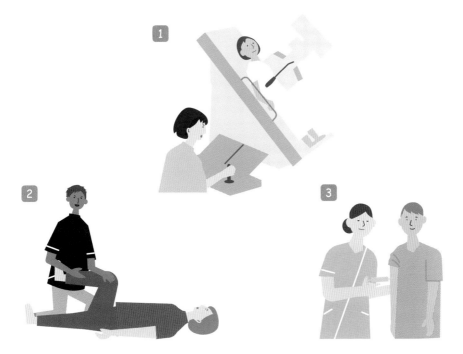

 What do you think?

Look at the following questions. Write down your opinion in response to each question. Share your opinions with the class, in small groups, or with your teacher.

1. A good way of making sure to give instructions clear and easy to understand is to say them in a way a child could understand them. How could this help you when speaking with patients?

2. What is "small talk," and why is that important in developing an open line of communication with patients?

3. What can you do to learn the skills needed to best communicate instructions to patients?

5

Basic instructions

Language corner

Below are some useful phrases you can use to give instructions to patients and their families. When giving instructions, be sure to use clear and simple sentences.

✅ In the waiting room

· Please tell me your full name and date of birth.
· Please fill out these forms.
· Please have a seat. Someone will call you soon.
· Please show me your health insurance card.

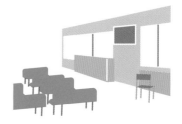

✅ In the examination room

· Take off your shirt and sit on the bed for me, please.
· Lie on your back, please.
· Take a deep breath and hold it. OK, breathe out.
· Raise your arms for me, please.

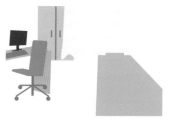

✅ Taking medication

· Take this (once, twice, three times) a day for two weeks.
· Don't drink alcohol while you are taking this medication.
· Please take the medicine after your meal.
· If you notice any side effects, contact the hospital.

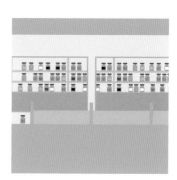

✅ On the ward

· How are you feeling today?
· I'm going to take your blood pressure. Please extend your right arm.
· Can you sit up for me, please?
· Turn to your side, please. Lie on your back. Turn to the other side for me, please.

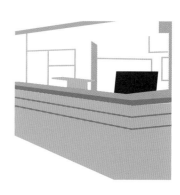

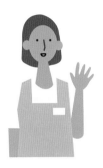

Name Susan Smith

Patient info 32-year-old female, hospitalized for the past 5 days with pneumonia

Comment Susan is an active person who enjoys playing tennis and hiking. She has a 7-year-old daughter. Her daughter is in the 2nd grade. Susan has been worrying about her daughter while she has been in the hospital. Susan has a husband who is doing his best to help, but he also has to work. Susan's friend is taking care of her daughter after school each day until her husband can pick her up. Susan talks to her husband and daughter by phone each evening. Susan is talkative and likes to chat with the nurses. She works as a store manager for a major retail chain. She may have gotten sick because of fatigue from her work and taking care of her home and family. Susan also has other interests such as jewelry making and baking. She promised to tell her cake recipe to the medical staff after she has been discharged from the hospital.

Chapter 6

Explaining treatment & results

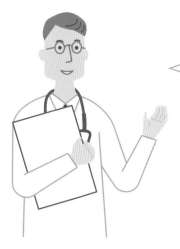

This treatment will improve your condition.

After completing medical tests, it is necessary for healthcare professionals to explain their findings and provide guidance on available therapies to their patients. It is more than just telling the patient the name of their illness and the drug used to treat it. It is about explaining how their current illness affects their life and why it may be necessary to make certain lifestyle changes to improve their health.

Listening practice 1

Listen to the following conversation between a doctor and a patient. Answer the following questions.

🔊 Track **6-1**

1. What were the results of the tests?

2. Why did the patient get tested?

3. What was the cause of the patient's problems?

4. Why did the doctor say there was no reason to be concerned?

5. Based on the dialogue, what do you think the prognosis is?

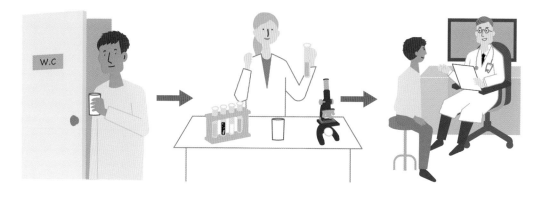

Listening practice 2

Listen to the following conversation between a doctor and a patient. Write the missing words and phrases, then answer the questions in the box below.

🔊 Track 6-2

Doctor: As I said before, what you have is a bacterial infection of the urinary tract. _____ are very effective at treating this type of problem.

Patient: Antibiotics?

Doctor: Yes, antibiotics are a type of drug that can kill unwanted _____ in the body.

Patient: I don't really like taking _____. Do these drugs have any _____ _____?

Doctor: Antibiotics are usually _____ _____, but sometimes side effects do occur. The most common ones include upset stomach, _____, and diarrhea. How do you feel about using this medicine?

Patient: That doesn't seem too bad. I think it's _____ _____ _____ if it will help me get better.

Doctor: In that case, I am going to write you a _____ for the drug Bactrim DS. For this medicine to be effective, you will need to take _____ _____ twice daily for three days.

Patient: I understand.

Doctor: If you have any _____ _____ _____, just give my office a call. I will be _____ to answer any questions you may have.

Patient: Thank you, Dr. Jones.

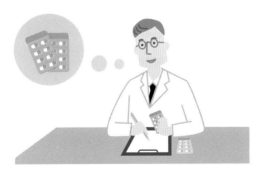

1. What are antibiotics?
2. What are the side effects of antibiotics?
3. How does the patient feel about taking the medicine?
4. What is a prescription?
5. How is the doctor being helpful?

Vocabulary

Below is a list of key vocabulary for this chapter. Translate each word or phrase into your native language.

1. rare _____

2. literacy _____

3. condition _____

4. (medical) test _____

5. positive (result) _____

6. negative (result) _____

7. prescription _____

8. dosage form _____

9. route of administration _____

10. (dosage) frequency _____

11. prognosis _____

12. abnormal _____

13. therapy _____

14. infection _____

15. inconclusive _____

16. disease _____

17. contagious _____

18. illness _____

19. pharmacy _____

20. side effect _____

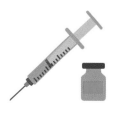

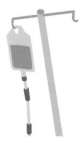
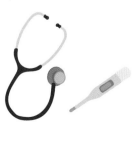

Crossword

Using the hints below, fill in the words to the puzzle.

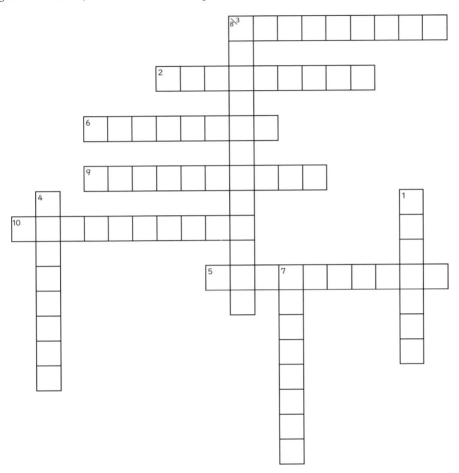

1. This is medical treatment for illness or injury.
2. This happens when viruses, bacteria, fungi, or parasites enter the human body and cause diseases.
3. This is the expected outcome of a disease, including whether it will improve, worsen, or stay the same over time.
4. This describes how much patients know about their disease.
5. This is the final shape the drug will take (pill, inhaler, injection etc.).
6. This is a retail store where drugs/medicine are sold.
7. This means that the body is functioning in a strange way or has something that should not be there.
8. These are written instructions by a doctor for a medication to be used by the patient at a pharmacy.
9. This means that a disease can be passed from one person to another.
10. This is a secondary and usually undesired effect of a drug.

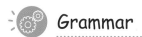 **Grammar**

Future tense

The future tense in English can be very useful when speaking to patients about their disease prognosis and also providing guidance on treatment. Here are two common ways to speak about the future in English.

▶ Will (simple future tense)

When do we use the simple future tense (phrases with the word "will")?

(1) To predict a future event or situation
   - Ex That drug **will** surely cause side effects if you take it with your other medication.
(2) To express a spontaneous decision (something that was not planned beforehand)
   - Ex It's hot, isn't it? I **will** open the window. (= I've just decided to open it at that time)
(3) When agreeing, refusing, or offering to do something, or when asking someone to do something
   - Ex **Will** you be able to come back next week for a follow-up appointment?

▶ Be going to

We also use "**be going to**" to say things about the future. However, "going to" and "will" have slightly different uses.

(1) To refer to our plans and intentions
   - Ex The doctor **is going to** perform an operation at 4 PM today. (= the doctor has a plan or appointment to perform an operation before the time of speaking)
(2) To make predictions based on present evidence. (= it is clear *now* that it is sure to happen.)
   - Ex You **are** probably **going to** experience some discomfort after the injection. (the injection → experience some discomfort)

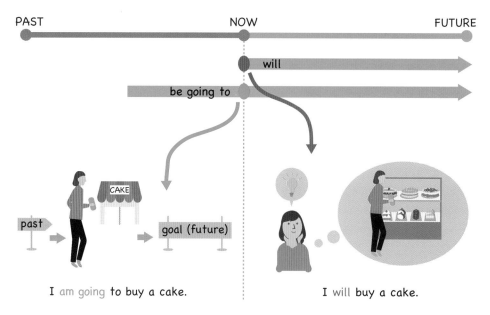

I am going to buy a cake.   I will buy a cake.

1 Fill in the blanks. Choose between "will" or "be going to." When using "be going to," remember to change the "be" verb to match the corresponding subject.

1. I think Dr. Miyake should look at this. I _____ call her now.

2. If you continue your current eating habits, you _____ experience health problems.

3. I _____ answer any questions you have.

4. According to the schedule, she _____ come in for an appointment next Friday.

5. I've made my decision. I _____ lose five kilograms this year.

2 Write sentences in the future tense using the following prompts.

1. Subject: The patient / Future tense verb: will

2. Subject: Dr. Kuramochi / Future tense verb: be going to

3. Future tense verb: will / Main verb: cause

4. Future tense verb: be going to / Main verb or object: have surgery

5. Subject: This medication / Main verb: lower

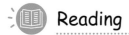 **Reading**

Read the following passage. Answer the questions in the box below.

Besides having a clear strategy for collecting diagnostically relevant information, the second most important job of healthcare professionals is explaining treatment and results. Below are a few things you should keep in mind.

✔ Meet one-on-one:

Interacting with patients one-on-one will make them feel more comfortable and allow them to ask questions. If you listen closely to their questions, you can measure their health literacy. Once you have a good estimate of their level of understanding, you can customize the way you communicate information to match it.

✔ Speak in simple English:

It is easy to forget your understanding of healthcare did not come easily. You have spent many years studying to achieve this level of knowledge. Your patients will probably not have had the same experience. While you may be able to speak the language of medicine, this language will be "foreign" to many of your patients. Therefore, you must use a language they can understand. Use only simple English when explaining illnesses and therapies.

✔ Give a physical demonstration:

In English, we have an expression, "monkey see, monkey do." This is a simple way of saying we learn by watching and imitating. Some therapies can be quite complicated, but even the most complicated treatments can be learned by patients when healthcare professionals give a physical demonstration. Try to use body language to communicate your message.

✔ Use the teach-back method:

Patients will often say they understand what they are told when, in reality, they do not. The teachback method is used to confirm whether or not a patient understands. After explaining an illness or treatment, ask the patient to repeat back to you, in their own words, what they have heard. If they cannot do this, then important information must be provided again in a way that is easier for the patient to understand.

✔ Provide written information:

Some patients are visual learners. For them, seeing what you explained in written form can significantly improve their understanding. Furthermore, giving the patient a copy of this information will allow them to reread your explanation at their own pace at home.

> **1.** What do you think will happen if you use a lot of medical words when talking to patients?
> **2.** What is the "teach-back" method and why is it important?
> **3.** Why is it a good idea to write down important information for your patients?

Speaking & writing

Look at the following questions. Write down your opinion in response to each question. Share your opinions with the class, in small groups, or with your teacher.

1. Telemedicine is becoming a more common way of interacting with patients. Do you think this will have a positive or negative effect on patient education? Why?

2. It takes time to effectively communicate results and treatment plans to patients. Doctors are already very busy. Are there any other healthcare professionals that can assist doctors in patient education? If so, who? In what way can they help?

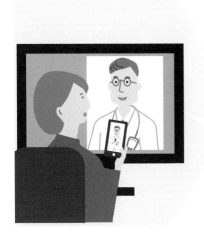

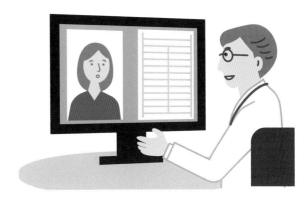

What do you think?

Look at the following questions. Write down your opinion in response to each question. Share your opinions with the class, in small groups, or with your teacher.

1. Health literacy plays an important part in whether a patient understands their disease and treatment plan. What can be done to improve health literacy in the general public?

2. As a healthcare professional, what can you do to help your patients understand their illness and treatment better?

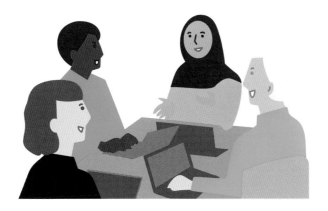

Language corner

Below are some phrases you can use when communicating in the clinical setting.

✅ Meet one-on-one

Useful phrases
· Thank you for coming in today.
· I have asked my staff not to disturb us.

Bad example
· This is my team of students and staff. We will all be interviewing you today. (not private)

✅ Speak in simple English

Useful phrases
· We will do some tests to check your heart.
· The X-ray shows that you have a tumor in your upper left lung.

Bad example
· The test results showed clear cell sarcoma on the right apex of the lung. (too technical)

✅ Give a physical demonstration

Useful phrases
· Hold your head back like this.
· Apply pressure to your arm like this.

Bad example
· Please turn your body so I can take a better X-ray. (too vague)

✅ Use the teach-back method

Useful phrases
· Can you tell me in your own words what we talked about today?
· In order to be sure that you understand, please explain it to me in your own words.

Bad example
· Did you understand? Prove it. What did I just say? (rude, attacking)

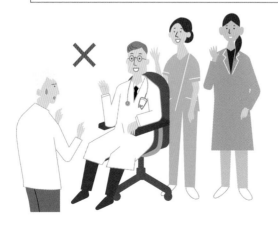
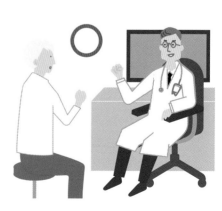

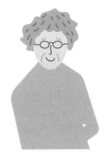

Name Beverly Barker

Patient info 86-year-old female with chronic respiratory conditions

Comment Recently, I have been having fever and difficulty breathing, so I promptly went to see the doctor. While speaking with the doctor, I got the distinct feeling that he was busy and did not have much time for me. He explained to me his thoughts on my current condition very quickly and with words I did not understand. I was confused and too embarrassed to tell him that I did not know what he was talking about. Seeing as he was in a hurry, I also did not want him to get frustrated with me if I asked too many questions. I left the doctor's office with the medicine that he recommended for the treatment of my illness, but I felt confused and uneasy. I still did not understand what was happening to me or how the medicine was going to help.

The medicine ended up resolving my problem, and I am grateful for my doctor's support. However, I think I would have been a lot less anxious if my doctor had taken a little more time to explain my condition and treatment to me in simple, plain language. Being sick is a scary experience for me. When I am sick, my body starts to feel and act differently than expected. In a way, I am scared because I feel a loss of control. If I understood my illness better, I feel like I would have more control over the situation, and this would help me to worry less.

7 How pain affects the patient

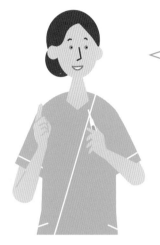

> The patient has had a headache for several days.

What is pain? Pain refers to physical suffering associated with bodily disorders, such as a disease or an injury, as well as mental or emotional distress. Pain affects us differently—some people have a high tolerance to pain, while others do not. Pain can also affect patients' mood and behavior. Healthcare professionals need to know how much the patient is suffering by asking about the location, intensity, or character of the pain.

Listening practice 1

Listen to the following conversation between a doctor and a patient. Choose the right words or phrases for each sentence.

🔊 Track 7-1

1. The patient has a (headache / stomachache).

2. The pain started about (2 / 3) days ago.

3. The level of her pain is (1 / 10).

4. She has the pain (only at night / all day).

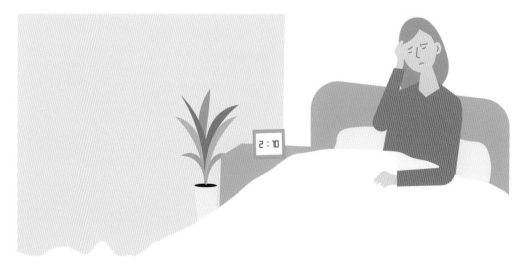

Listening practice 2

Listen to the following conversation between a doctor and a patient. Complete the notes below. If there is no corresponding answer, leave the answer space blank.

🔊 Track 7-2

Onset of the pain: _____

Palliation & provocation: _____

Quality of the pain: _____

Region & radiation: _____

Severity of the pain (1 to 10): _____

Timing of the pain: _____

🔊 Track 7-3

Onset of the pain: _____

Palliation & provocation: _____

Quality of the pain: _____

Region & radiation: _____

Severity of the pain (1 to 10): _____

Timing of the pain: _____

🔊 Track 7-4

Onset of the pain: _____

Palliation & provocation: _____

Quality of the pain: _____

Region & radiation: _____

Severity of the pain (1 to 10): _____

Timing of the pain: _____

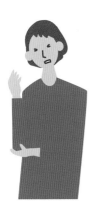
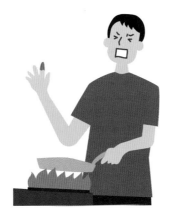
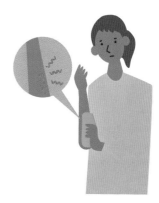

7

How pain affects the patient

Vocabulary

Below is a list of key vocabulary for this chapter. Translate each word or phrase into your native language.

1. suffer　_____
2. distress　_____
3. intensity　_____
4. joint　_____
5. psychological　_____
6. mild　_____
7. moderate　_____
8. severe　_____
9. constant　_____
10. intermittent　_____
11. acute　_____
12. chronic　_____
13. sharp　_____
14. cramping　_____
15. tingling　_____
16. numb　_____
17. itchy　_____
18. sore　_____
19. tolerance　_____
20. ache　_____

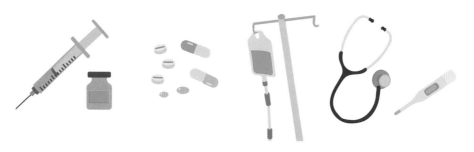

Word maze

Help the patient find the physical therapy department. Start from the center of the maze. Read the clues written below to find the correct path to the physical therapy department. Each word must be connected to the next word by a straight line. Which room is it in? Follow the line to find the answer.

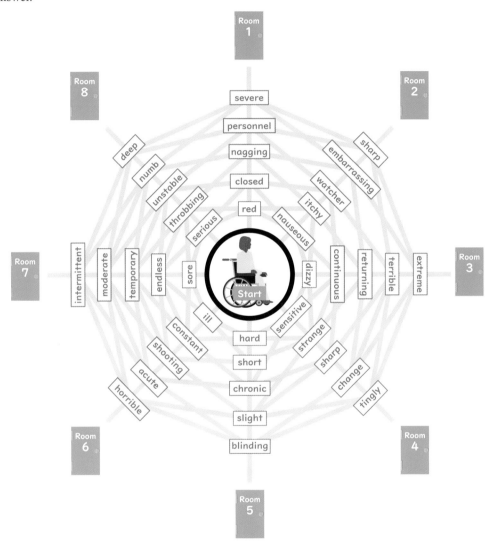

1. A word that means slightly painful.
2. A word that means something is continually occurring.
3. A word that means pain that lasts for more than six months.
4. A word that means pain that lasts less than six months.
5. A word that means the pain is not severe and can be ignored.
6. A word that means the pain comes and goes.
7. A word that means loss of feeling or having a tingling sensation.
8. A word that means extremely bad.

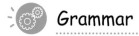 Grammar

Perfect tense

▶ **The present perfect tense (have + past participle)**

(1) The present perfect tense is used to express an action that started in the past and continues now.

    Ex I **have had** a headache for several days.

    Ex How long **have** you **had** the symptoms?

(2) It is also used to talk about experiences.

    Ex I **have** never **been** to Hawaii. (in my life)

    Ex The patient **has had** two operations on his knee.

(3) The present perfect tense describes a present action that began in the past and is completed in the present.

    Ex She **has washed** her hands and is ready to eat.

    Ex The doctor **has finished** preparing for surgery.

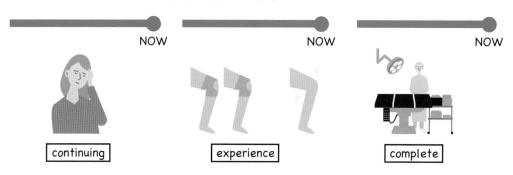

▶ **The past perfect tense (had + past participle)**

(1) The past perfect tense describes an action that began in the past and was completed in the past before something else occurred.

    Ex He **had finished** his treatment before his family arrived. (Here, the treatment began and ended before the family arrived.)

(2) It can also be used to describe an experience (or a lack of an experience) before a certain point in the past.

    Ex I **had** never **tried** sushi until I came to Japan. (In this situation, the speaker tried sushi for the first time when she came to Japan at a point in the past.)

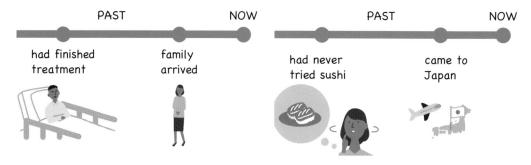

▶ The present perfect continuous tense (have + been + present participle)

There is also the present perfect continuous tense, which describes something that began in the past and is still happening frequently in the present.

> **Ex** I have been having dizziness recently. (= I'm still having dizziness.)
>
> **Ex** I have been coughing all the time since Tuesday.

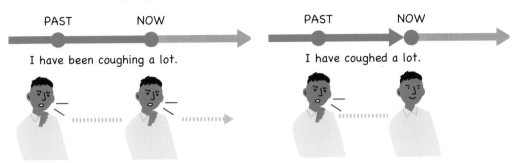

PAST   NOW   PAST   NOW

I have been coughing a lot.   I have coughed a lot.

> ### 💡 Key Points
>
> The present perfect tense and present perfect continuous tense have slightly different uses. Sentences in the present perfect tense generally focus on a result or a completed action. "I've read the book" means that the person has finished reading the book. On the other hand, sentences in the present perfect continuous tense focus on the activity itself or something that's still going on. "I've been reading the book," a present perfect continuous sentence, means that the person started reading the book earlier and is still reading the book.

Complete the sentences below with the verbs written in parentheses. Use the proper perfect tense for each sentence.

1. He _____ _____ (talk) to several specialists about his problem, but nobody knows why he is sick.

2. I _____ _____ _____ (feel) some discomfort in my neck since this morning.

3. Ken _____ _____ (promise) to stay with his younger brother, so he couldn't come to the party.

4. The patient _____ _____ (recover) completely by the time he left the hospital.

5. The doctor _____ _____ (examine) thousands of patients over her career.

Reading

Read the following passage. Circle whether each is true or false in the box below.

When we talk about pain, we tend to pay attention to physical pain, such as headaches, stomachaches, and backaches. However, all of us have experienced another type of pain, which is "emotional pain." Unlike physical pain that can be seen by bleeding wounds or broken legs, emotional pain is something that is hard to see from outside. In this chapter, we will focus on two types of emotional pain. The first is sadness. As the idiom "die of a broken heart" suggests, sadness can negatively affect our health. A person who lost his or her spouse, for example, might feel as if they have lost the will to live. Others who have been diagnosed with a serious illness might feel there is no hope for the future and give up fighting to become healthy.

The other common type of emotional pain is anger. Patients might express their anger for various reasons. Some may get angry because they had to wait too long. Others may become angry because they feel the treatment they got from healthcare professionals was not what they wanted. Some might be enduring horrible pain, which may be affecting their emotions.

Sadness and anger are just two of the many types of emotional pains that healthcare workers should pay attention to. Once they recognize emotional pain in their patients, healthcare workers should think about ways of handling the situation so that they can do their best to care for their patients. Unless you are a psychologist, you do not need to diagnose the cause of your patients' emotional pain or offer specific treatment. Instead, you should be aware of the emotional state of your patients and let them release their emotional pain if they need to. It is important that patients feel that healthcare workers recognize their emotional states and empathize with them. On the other hand, there might be some patients who do not want to share their emotional pain with healthcare professionals. In that case, you should not force them. Instead, give the patients some time before you move onto the next process.

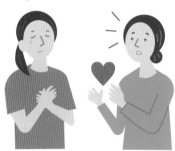

1. It is easy to recognize emotional pain from the outside. (T / F)
2. When people feel sad, the degree of sadness is different depending on each person.
(T / F)
3. Some people are angry because they suffer from severe pain. (T / F)
4. It is important for all doctors to diagnose the cause of the patients' emotional pain.
(T / F)
5. When patients are in a state of emotional distress, it sometimes works to give them some time. (T / F)

Speaking & writing

Write down all the types of pain you can think of. If you don't know the words in English, check with your dictionary.

Ex *headache, backache, stomachache, toothache*

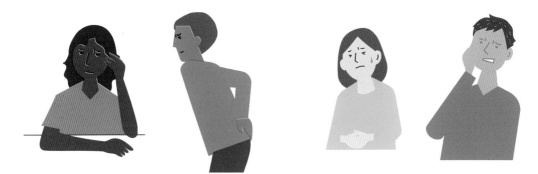

 ## What do you think?

Look at the following questions. Write down your opinion in response to each question. Share your opinions with the class, in small groups, or with your teacher.

1. Write down your story about emotional pain. Try to remember as many details as you can. You should especially write down how you felt, how this feeling affected your behavior, how you were able to overcome this situation, and how overcoming your emotional pain changed your behavior.

2. Share your story with several members of your class. You will also be asked to listen to other people's stories. By sharing your story, you will get some sense of how patients feel when they are sharing their stories. Don't forget to use active listening.

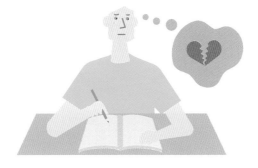

Language corner

Pain is one of the most common symptoms. For that reason, you will have many opportunities to talk to your patients about pain. Below are some helpful phrases you can use.

✅ Describing pain

It is important that you learn various ways to describe pain. The type of pain can tell healthcare professionals a lot about what's going on with the patient.

- **An** aching **pain** is one that is not too severe but is continuous.
- **A** throbbing **pain** is stronger than an aching pain. It feels like it beats with a strong pulse or rhythm.
- **A** sharp **pain** is a sudden and strong burst of pain, such as a sudden chest pain.
- **A** burning **pain** can feel like skin or muscles are being heated up. Rashes are often described as having a burning pain.
- **A** cramp **or cramping pain** is caused by a sudden tightening of muscles.

> **Useful phrases**
> · How does the rash feel? Is it itchy, burning, or painful?

✅ Pain scale

It is challenging for healthcare professionals to know how much pain patients are suffering from. It is also challenging for the patients to describe their pain to the doctor. In order to measure the pain as accurately as possible, a numeric pain scale is used. The pain scale is a simple way to rate the intensity of the pain. Patients rate their pain on a scale of 1 (very mild pain) to 10 (the most severe pain).

> **Useful phrases**
> · On a scale of one to ten, one being a very mild pain and ten being unbearable, how would you rate your pain?

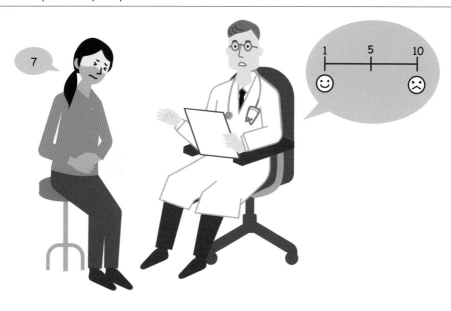

Anesthesia

Anesthesia is medicine that is used to prevent or reduce the feeling of pain when people are having surgery or other painful procedures. According to the World Federation of Societies of Anesthesiologists (WFSA), the first public demonstration of anesthesia took place in 1846, at Massachusetts General Hospital in Boston. Before anesthesia was in practice, surgery had been done as a last resort. Few people survived. After the demonstration took place, various types of anesthesia were tested. Since then, the field of anesthesiology has undergone a great advancement. At present, there are different types of anesthesia; general and local. General anesthesia makes patients completely unconscious. They don't feel any pain during an operation. The local anesthesia doesn't make the patients fall asleep. Instead it numbs the parts of the body where patients might feel pain. Local anesthesia is used for stitches, dental work, or minor surgeries.

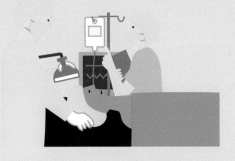

 Homework

Think of why it is important for healthcare professionals to reflect on their own experiences of pain.

8 Nutrition

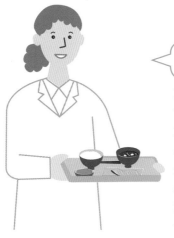

Are you eating well?

Food is more than just nourishment. People across the globe bond over food. Food is the foundation of life—it provides health, makes life more fun, and connects people from different cultures. Although eating can be a joy, the consumption of food is also connected to health problems such as diabetes and eating disorders. In order to understand the importance of a healthy and satisfying diet, this chapter examines the ways in which people perceive food culture, food health, and nutrition.

Listening practice 1

Listen to the following track. Answer true or false to the following questions.

🔊 Track 8-1

1. The first line of defense in preventing disease is good medicine.　　　(T / F)

2. Food contains things the body needs to function properly.　　　(T / F)

3. Taking supplements is just as effective as eating properly.　　　(T / F)

4. Eating too many processed foods and foods high in sugar or salt is OK if they have lots of vitamins.　　　(T / F)

5. Recommendations for eating well should be included in treatment plans.　　　(T / F)

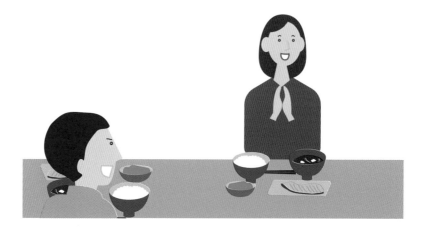

Listening practice 2

Listen to a healthcare professional explain a patient's case report. Write in the missing words and phrases, then answer the questions in the box below.

🔊 Track 8-2

The patient is a _____ _____ who suffers from an _____ _____ called bulimia nervosa, which is sometimes called bulimia for short. This eating disorder is _____ by the patient's habit of binge eating and purging. _____ means getting rid of food that has been consumed. It typically happens by vomiting or _____ laxatives. In our patient's case, she purges by vomiting. The effects of bulimia include dehydration, _____ problems, low _____ pressure, _____ to the esophagus, hormonal _____, tooth decay, and electrolyte imbalance. Electrolytes are _____ such as minerals and salts that help conduct _____ signals in the body. People suffering from bulimia often have an imbalance of potassium, sodium, and other electrolytes. Electrolyte imbalance is usually caused by the _____ ____ _____ during purging. It is important that we pay close attention to our patient's _____ states, as bulimic patients often _____ from anxiety, depression, self-harm, and low self-image. We will be working with nutritionists and psychologists to help get this patient back to a _____ state. We will also be working closely with the _____ staff to come up with a daily care plan.

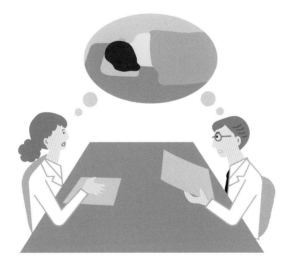

1. Is the patient a man or a woman?
2. What is bulimia nervosa?
3. How does bulimia nervosa affect the patient's physical condition?
4. What are the nutritional effects of bulimia nervosa?
5. How does bulimia nervosa affect the patient's psychological condition?

Vocabulary

Below is a list of key vocabulary for this chapter. Translate each word or phrase into your native language.

1. diet _____

2. nutrient _____

3. allergy _____

4. supplement _____

5. malnutrition _____

6. eating disorder _____

7. composition _____

8. abuse _____

9. consumption _____

10. addiction _____

11. metabolism _____

12. intake _____

13. mineral _____

14. processed _____

15. desirable _____

16. food intolerance _____

17. quantity _____

18. habit _____

19. comfort food _____

20. contamination _____

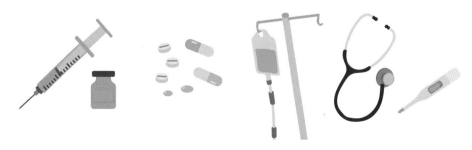

Match illustrations and words or phrases

Look at the illustrations below. Choose the word or phrase that matches the illustration.

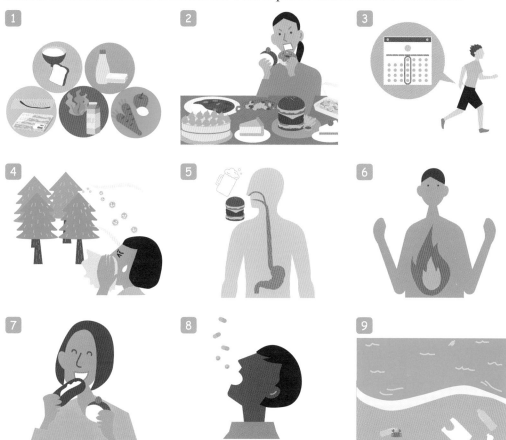

comfort food / contamination / intake / allergy / habit /
metabolism / nutrient / abuse / eating disorder

	Words / Phrases		Words / Phrases		Words / Phrases
1.		4.		7.	
2.		5.		8.	
3.		6.		9.	

Nutrition

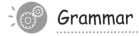 **Grammar**

Continuous tenses

▸ **The present continuous (be + present participle, or the "-ing" form of the verb) is used:**

(1) When an action is happening at that moment

Ex Ken **is playing** the piano. (Here, Ken is playing the piano now.)

Ex The patient **is waiting** to see you, Doctor. (The patient is actually waiting at that moment.)

(2) To describe temporary or new habits

Ex He's **drinking** a lot these days.

(3) To describe habits that are regular

Ex She **is always singing** in the shower.

(4) To describe future plans

Ex I'm **going** to Hokkaido for summer vacation.

Ex I'm **undergoing** surgery next Thursday.

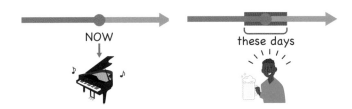

▸ **The past continuous (was/were + present participle, or the "-ing" form of the verb) is used:**

(1) When we want to show that something continued over time in the past

Ex They **were making** noise for three hours yesterday.

(2) When something was happening before another action

Ex They **were watching** TV when I left the room.

(3) When something happened continuously before and after a specific time

Ex At 5 PM, I **was doing** my homework. (I started before 5 PM and continued after 5 PM.)

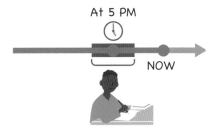

▶ **Verbs that are rarely used in continuous forms**

There are some verbs that we rarely use in the continuous form. Here are some examples:

belong × I am belonging to the soccer club./○ I belong to the soccer club.

want × She is wanting a second opinion./○ She wants a second opinion.

need × I am needing some help./○ I need some help.

 Key Points

The two main present continuous tenses—the present continuous and present perfect continuous—can be confusing. To make sure you use them correctly, just remember that the present continuous shows that an action is happening right now. For example, "She's waiting for the train" simply means that the person is waiting at this moment. The present perfect continuous, or "have + been + present participle," is often used to show that the action started in the past and is still continuing. Sentences like "She has been waiting for the train" or "She has been waiting for the train for 10 minutes" indicate that the person started waiting some time ago, so they emphasize a duration.

Circle the correct words in the sentence.

1. He (gets / is getting) enough nutrients lately.

2. I (am believing / believe) that the doctor told me the truth.

3. The patient (adores / is adoring) her doctor.

4. He (is walking / walks) to the station now.

5. Mary wanted to be a doctor when she (was / was being) a girl.

6. The dog and his owner (are resembling / resemble) each other.

7. I (visit / am visiting) the university for a lecture next week.

8. (Do you understand / Are you understanding) the nurse's instructions?

9. She (takes more supplements / is taking more supplements) now than she was a week ago.

10. The patient (has / is having) an allergy to penicillin.

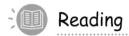 ## Reading

Read the following passage. Answer the questions in the box below.

Food is the most essential ingredient for health. There is an expression in English that goes, "You are what you eat." That means our bodies are made of the nutrients we consume. Proteins help to build our muscles; calcium helps to make bones; and vitamins and minerals help to keep the systems of our bodies running smoothly. If our nutritional balance is bad, it can have a negative impact on our health. Some common diseases that are directly connected to food are cancer, heart disease, diabetes, and hypertension. In ancient times, sailors would go for months without fresh fruits and vegetables. As a result, they would often get a disease called scurvy. The symptoms are joint pain, blood spots under the skin, loose teeth, extremely bad breath, and extreme weakness. Scurvy could even cause death. All of this was because of a lack of vitamin C.

Food is also important to patients' psychological well-being. People are comfortable eating food that they know. There is another expression in English, "comfort food," which is food that makes you feel safe and comfortable or food that brings back memories of childhood. If patients are far away from their country, comfort food can also bring back feelings of home. On the other hand, if food is too different from what the patient is used to, or if the food does not seem delicious or desirable, then patients may have a problem getting proper nutrition because they may refuse to eat. Patients may also feel unnecessary stress, which could interfere with the healing process.

One of the things that most healthcare institutions are responsible for is patients' quality of life. Remember that a balanced menu is also part of the patient's quality of life. Patients should be able to get food that is nutritionally balanced and also psychologically balanced. Although it may not have much nutritional value, a cookie, some soda, or a piece of candy could go a long way to helping your patients feel at ease.

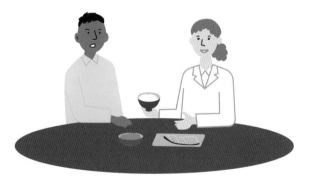

1. What are the two essential functions of food?
2. What are the common diseases caused by malnutrition?
3. What should you consider when making food choices?

Speaking & writing

Look at the following questions about comfort food. Write down your opinion in response to each question. Share your opinions with the class, in small groups, or with your teacher.

1. What is your favorite food? Do you have any special memories attached to it?

2. In your culture, are there any special dishes that people make or eat to celebrate special occasions? What are they?

3. Is there any food you crave when you are tired? What about to relieve stress?

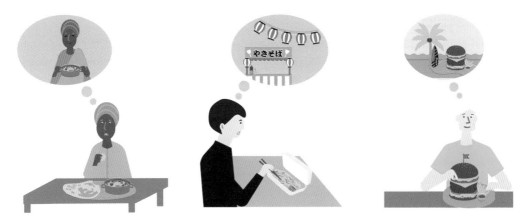

 ## What do you think?

Look at the following questions. Write down your opinion in response to each question. Share your opinions with the class, in small groups, or with your teacher.

1. How can we teach and encourage children to have healthy eating habits?

2. Some countries put taxes on unhealthy foods. Is this a good idea?

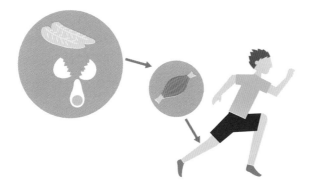

Language corner

Nutrition is a very important part of healthcare. Below are some useful sentences that you can use to talk to your future patients about nutrition.

Health benefits of food

Food gives us the power to fight disease and the power to heal. It is the fuel we use to operate our bodies. It is very important that your patients maintain a balanced and nutritious diet.

> **Useful phrases**
> · Eating a nutritious and healthy meal will help you maintain your health.
> · Please avoid eating too many carbohydrates because they can cause weight gain.
> · Please limit your sugar intake to one sweet thing a day.

Safety

Food safety is a top priority in healthcare institutions. It is also a top priority for patients who are being cared for at home. Below are some useful phrases and sentences that you can use to talk about food safety.

> **Useful phrases**
> · Be sure to keep perishable foods in the refrigerator.
> · Check the expiration date on foods such as eggs, milk, and meat.
> · To avoid food poisoning, do not eat food that has been in the refrigerator for more than three days.

Preparing and serving food

How food is prepared may also have an impact on health. Below are some useful sentences you can use to talk about food preparation with your patients.

> **Useful phrases**
> · Sauteing meat and vegetables is much healthier than deep frying.
> · Raw vegetables contain the most nutrition.
> · Cooking at home is a great way to control your sodium intake and your budget.

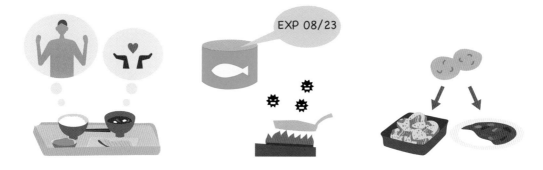

Sports dietitian

Dr. Uchino, a pioneer in the field of sports nutrition, works with Paralympians. Athletes who train at the highest level follow specific eating plans and precise training methods to meet the high physical demands of competitive sports. Dietary restrictions can cause serious stress that may lead to poor performance. For Paralympic athletes whose events require strict weight control, dietitians must pay attention not only to their nutritional intake but also to their mental state. Working for

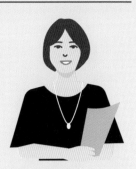

Paralympians also poses special challenges. The first athlete Dr. Uchino worked with said that he "couldn't sweat." He had an injury that impacted his autonomic nervous system and made it impossible for him to perspire. In order to make sure the athlete drank enough water and maintained adequate body temperature control, Dr. Uchino suggested he put crushed ice in his mouth to hydrate himself while lowering his body temperature. Experiences like these gave Dr. Uchino deep insights into patient care and professionalism. "It all starts with individual attention through careful communication," Dr. Uchino says. "As with everything, it takes a team to achieve great results."

 ## Homework

Log your food intake for a week. After you have completed your food log, analyze it and think about the following questions:

1. Are there any habits or patterns in your diet?
2. Are there any nutritional imbalances in your diet?
3. Which dishes brought you joy, and which did not?

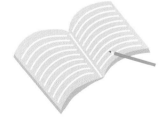

9 Inpatients

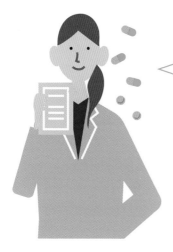

This is the pill which will relieve your pain.

Patients can be hospitalized for various reasons, some for several days, and some for longer. In addition to health concerns, leaving home for a long period can cause worries about their families and homes. Being with a large group of unfamiliar people can further stress the patient. Through good communication practices, healthcare professionals can ease their patients' anxiety by showing them that they are being heard and understood.

Listening practice 1

Listen to the following conversation between a doctor and a patient. Choose the right word or phrase for each sentence.

🔊 Track 9-1

1. The patient feels (dizzy / hungry).
2. The doctor explains that the patient's symptoms are (surprising / not surprising).
3. According to the medical chart, the surgery was (successful / not successful).
4. The patient wants to see her (parents / husband).
5. The husband was finally able to relax after (speaking to the doctor / the operation was finished).

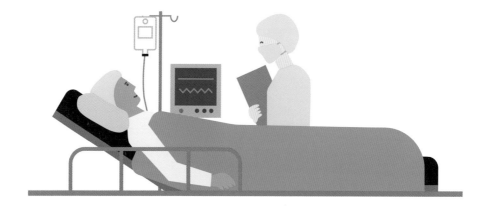

Listen to the following conversation between a nurse and a patient. Write the missing words and phrases.

◀)) Track 9-2

Nurse: Mr. Wilson, your surgery is _____ for 11 o'clock tomorrow morning. Do you have any _____ about your surgery?

Patient: I'm worried that the surgery may be painful.

Nurse: You will not feel any pain during the surgery because we will use _____ _____. But you might feel a little pain as the anesthetic _____ _____. If that happens, we can give you some pain _____.

Patient: I'm happy to hear that. By the way, what time are the _____ _____ ? My daughter will come to visit me later.

Nurse: From 10 AM to 6 PM. We can prepare a private space for you. If you need it, feel free to tell us.

Patient: Thank you very much. When will I be able to go home? I would like to be _____ as soon as possible.

Nurse: It depends on your post-operative _____. When the doctor comes on his _____, you can ask him for more information.

Patient: I see. Thank you.

◀)) Track 9-3

Nurse: Mr. Brown, let me change the _____. I will _____ your clothes.

Patient: Yes, please do it gently.

Nurse: Do you have any pain around the _____?

Patient: Yes, it's still a little painful. When will it get better?

Nurse: It's getting better and better, so you don't have to _____. I recommend practicing walking every day for _____. If you practice a lot, you will be able to move smoothly.

Patient: I'm worried about practicing _____. Can somebody help me?

Nurse: Of course, we will support you. It seems you are worried about your stay in the hospital. If so, please know that not only doctors and nurses but all of our healthcare _____ will work together so you can safely be discharged. For a quick recovery, it is very important that you follow the guidance of the _____ _____.

Patient: I am very _____ to hear that. I'll try.

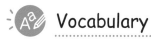 Vocabulary

Below is a list of key vocabulary for this chapter. Translate each word or phrase into your native language.

1. diagnose _____

2. hospitalization _____

3. discharge _____

4. inpatient _____

5. visiting hours _____

6. consent form _____

7. anesthesia _____

8. wear off _____

9. medical chart _____

10. bed bath _____

11. incision _____

12. complication _____

13. preoperative _____

14. well-being _____

15. IV drip (intravenous drip) _____

16. rehabilitation _____

17. reassure _____

18. outpatient _____

19. undo _____

20. admit _____

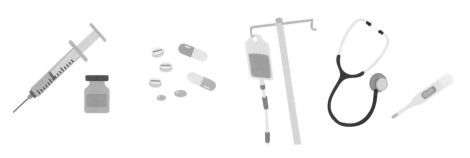

Word search

Find the words that are written in the list below. Words can be across, up and down, or diagonal.

```
B  U  Z  P  D  J  Q  Z  K  N  R  E  A  S  S  U  R  E  P  R
A  C  A  D  T  U  G  O  I  N  C  I  S  I  O  N  A  C  R  I
Z  C  O  C  G  W  M  X  L  M  O  T  N  H  J  U  Z  C  E  M
A  D  M  I  T  Z  P  I  V  O  M  Z  J  O  X  N  H  B  O  T
T  R  R  W  A  R  X  G  Z  B  P  B  N  M  S  D  S  I  P  K
Q  P  E  A  G  Z  Q  H  Z  R  L  M  A  P  B  O  I  N  E  B
I  U  H  O  S  P  I  T  A  L  I  Z  A  T  I  O  N  I  R  E
V  V  A  A  W  E  F  I  B  H  C  D  A  D  K  J  E  W  A  D
D  A  B  G  D  B  R  A  A  G  A  R  I  Q  C  K  K  P  T  B
R  F  I  B  G  M  H  N  W  I  T  R  C  A  X  K  F  X  I  A
I  A  L  Q  N  W  I  E  Z  X  I  F  H  P  G  D  G  R  V  T
P  R  I  H  J  E  X  S  Z  W  O  R  D  L  B  N  O  T  E  H
V  B  T  P  W  A  Y  T  S  Z  N  L  F  S  I  F  O  T  T  Y
G  C  A  R  A  R  F  H  G  I  S  O  D  M  L  I  K  S  G  M
S  V  T  W  P  O  Z  E  Z  P  O  E  T  F  W  Z  T  K  E  I
O  Y  I  A  Z  F  N  S  W  H  I  N  P  A  T  I  E  N  T  P
C  F  O  R  I  F  U  I  J  O  M  L  S  Y  W  D  J  S  O  C
C  V  N  W  B  Q  W  A  M  Q  Y  C  Z  C  N  I  Y  Z  U  R
O  D  L  Z  O  U  T  P  A  T  I  E  N  T  R  S  A  P  D  S
U  O  C  G  D  J  G  D  I  S  C  H  A  R  G  E  W  V  T  G
```

DIAGNOSE	HOSPITALIZATION	DISCHARGE	INPATIENT
ANESTHESIA	WEAR OFF	BED BATH	INCISION
COMPLICATION	PREOPERATIVE	IV DRIP	REHABILITATION
REASSURE	OUTPATIENT	UNDO	ADMIT

Grammar

Relative clauses

When you want to give more information about a **noun**, the simplest way is to put an adjective before it ("beautiful **flowers**"). However, there are many times when you want to give more information than one adjective can provide. Relative clauses are very useful for giving additional information about a noun (an antecedent).

Unlike an adjective, a relative clause comes after the noun it describes.
The basic pattern goes like this: **noun** (antecedent) + **relative pronoun** + additional information about the antecedent.

The relative pronoun is the link between the noun and the additional information. It needs to match the antecedent. Here are some common relative pronouns:

▸ Who
Use **who** when a person is the antecedent.
Ex **The girl** (antecedent) **who** is standing at the entrance of the classroom is Alice.
Ex She will go to the movies next week with **the man who** just came in.
Ex This is **the nurse who** will take care of you.

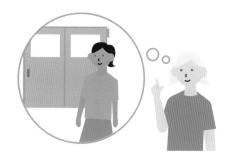

▸ Which
Use **which** when a thing or animal is the antecedent.
Ex **The pill which** will relieve your pain.
Ex **The dog which** normally barks all the time is quiet this morning.

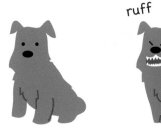

ruff ruff

▶ When

Use **when** if the antecedent is a word or phrase indicating time.

[Ex] **The day when** you arrived in New York was sunny and very hot.

[Ex] 1776 is **the year when** the United States became independent.

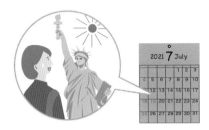

▶ Where

Use **where** when a place, situation, or position is the antecedent.

[Ex] This is **the hotel where** the great musician often stayed.

[Ex] Can you give me some more information about **the hospital room where** I'll be staying?

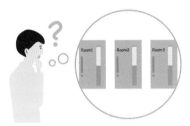

Fill in the blanks with the missing words. Choose from the words below.

who / which / when / where

1. We were very busy the year _____ our son was born.

2. The person _____ was involved in the accident was admitted to the hospital.

3. This is the medication _____ my doctor prescribed.

4. Could you tell me the name of the department _____ Dr. Takahata works?

5. That was the moment _____ I decided to become a doctor.

6. The anesthesia _____ you receive before the operation will wear off in a few hours.

7. I'm looking for the room _____ my father is doing rehabilitation.

8. The medical chart contained a lot of information _____ the nurse copied down.

9. Could you give me the name of the doctor _____ diagnosed you?

10. Doctors perform surgery only on patients _____ have signed the required consent form.

Reading

Read the following passage. Answer the questions in the box below.

It is a common mistake to think of bedside manner only as the way healthcare professionals behave when they are at the patients' bedside. In truth, bedside manner is about how healthcare professionals behave when they are in front of their patients. It includes interactions in a clinic, office, waiting room, or any place where there is an interaction between healthcare workers and their patients. It's not just about communication on the ward. Bedside manner has four major components. They are verbal communication, nonverbal communication, professionalism, and attitude.

Verbal communication refers to spoken language. It is the words you use to talk to your patients. You should always speak to them in a way that is polite and professional. As much as possible, you should also remember to use active listening skills. How you speak to a patient determines whether or not you have good bedside manner. You should always speak to patients in a way that shows basic respect regardless of their nationality, social status, physical condition, age, or gender.

Nonverbal communication is often overlooked, but it is an important part of bedside manner. Nonverbal communication is how we communicate with people using our body language instead of our words. This includes having good eye contact, good posture, appropriate facial expressions, and a confident appearance. Bad posture and other negative nonverbal communication can have a negative impact on your ability to build rapport.

Professionalism is at the heart of good bedside manner. It's more than just how you behave; professionalism is about your ability to see yourself as a professional healthcare provider. It is about behaving in a way that is appropriate to your profession. As a professional, you must see the patient as a human being in need of assistance or care and respect the patients' cultural or lifestyle differences.

Of course, all of these are tied together with a proper attitude. You should always speak to the patient with an attitude that shows empathy and caring. You should never speak to patients in a way that makes them feel as if they are not important to you.

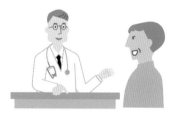

1. Please describe in your own words what bedside manner means.
2. Please describe in your own words what professionalism means.
3. What do you think is the effect of bad bedside manner?
4. How does nonverbal communication affect bedside manner?
5. Has your understanding of bedside manner changed after reading the text? If so, please explain how it has changed.

Speaking & writing

Look at the following questions. Write down your opinion in response to each question. Share your opinions with the class, in small groups, or with your teacher.

Imagine that you have to be admitted to the hospital for several weeks. What do you think your concerns will be?

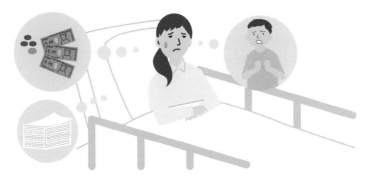

 ## What do you think?

Look at the following questions. Write down your opinion in response to each question. Share your opinions with the class, in small groups, or with your teacher.

1. What might cause patients to feel nervous before surgery?
2. What should you do for your patients to help them get rid of their anxiety?
3. What do you think you should do with patients who are not willing to do physical therapy after surgery?
4. What do you think patients feel anxious about while in the hospital? How can you encourage them in such a situation?

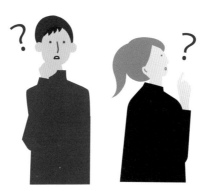

Language corner

Good bedside manner requires you to pay special attention to your patients through verbal and nonverbal communication. It also requires you to be professional and courteous at all times. Below are some sentences that you can use to help you have good bedside manner.

✅ Checking in on a patient

- How are you feeling today?
- Have there been any changes since I saw you last?
- Have you been taking the medication?
- I see you're doing much better today. That's great.
- Has your appetite come back?

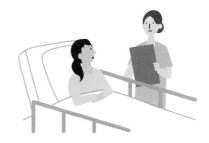

✅ Showing empathy

- I can see that you're worried.
- This must be a frustrating time for you.
- It's understandable that you feel anxious right now.
- I'm sorry to hear that.
- Thank you for sharing your feelings with me.

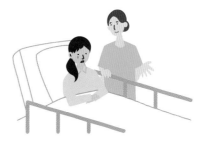

✅ Offering support and reassurance

- We will do our best to help you get through this difficult time.
- There are many treatment options available.
- I am here for you, so feel free to contact me anytime.
- We have assigned the best team of healthcare professionals to your case.
- The test results look hopeful.

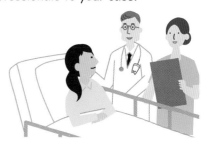

The first Japanese nurse

The concept of nursing as a career first appeared in Japan in the 1800s. Until then, Japanese doctors were unfamiliar with the term. Instead, the Japanese word kanbyonin was used to describe those who cared for the sick and the poor. Although *kanbyonin* have been around since ancient times, the profession had not been well established. There were no formal training methods, so anyone could become a *kanbyonin*. The Japanese government usually hired them. They were not seen as healthcare professionals. Instead, they were seen as servants. As more Japanese doctors returned to Japan from Britain and the US, the concept of nursing began to spread. Doctors began looking for *kanbyonin*, who had the skill to take care of patients and also had social and political influence. One woman stood out above the rest. Her name was Kane Sugimoto. She gained a reputation among doctors for her talent in caring for surgical cases. She was also known for her professionalism and respectable personality. In 1872, when Takanaka Sato founded Juntendo Hospital, he asked Kane Sugimoto to be his chief nurse. Today, she is considered to be the first nurse of note in Japan.

 Homework

Think of a time when you or someone you know was hospitalized. How did it feel and what were the challenges?

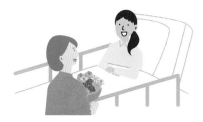

10 Breaking bad news

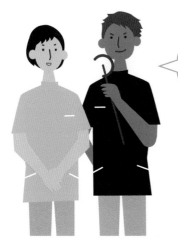

> Your test results look good, but I think we should be cautious.

Learning how to break bad news is an important part of learning how to be a good healthcare professional. Learning to break bad news the right way will help reduce stress for you and your patients. In this chapter, we will learn the SPIKES protocol. SPIKES is a widely used set of procedures for breaking bad news. By following the SPIKES protocol, healthcare professionals can increase their confidence when they have to disclose unfavorable medical information to their patients.

Listening practice 1

Listen to the following conversation between a new staff member and a senior staff member. Answer the following questions.

🔊 Track 10-1

1. What did the new staff member ask the senior staff member?

2. What did the senior staff member say about the importance of behavior?

3. What specific advice did the senior staff member give about posture?

4. Why do you think the new staff member asked the senior staff member for advice?

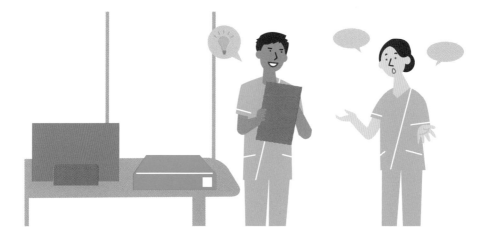

Language corner

Healthcare providers must be especially careful when delivering bad news. The way it is delivered can have a significant impact on future treatment. The SPIKES protocol is a step-by-step procedure for breaking bad news.

Step 1 : Setting

Make sure that you are uninterrupted and that your focus is on the patient.

> **Useful phrases**   We won't be interrupted. You have my complete attention.

Step 2 : Perception of condition/seriousness

It is important to have patients explain to you what they understand about their condition. This will help you to know what information to give and how to give it. This also gives you an opportunity to clear up any misunderstandings.

> **Useful phrases**   Please describe to me what you think is going on with you now.

Step 3 : Invitation from the patient to give information

Before delivering bad news, it's essential to make sure that the patient is ready to receive it. You must ask for permission. This important step cannot be skipped.

> **Useful phrases**   I have the test results for you. Would you like to hear them now, even if it's bad news, or would you prefer to have a family member with you?

Step 4 : Knowledge: giving medical facts

After you have been given permission to share the bad news, it is meaningful to use clear, easy-to-understand language to describe the health findings, prognosis, and treatment.

> **Useful phrases**   The test results have come back. Unfortunately, I do not have good news for you. The MRI showed there is a tumor in the front part of your brain. We must do further testing to understand the nature of the tumor and how to treat it.

Step 5 : Explore emotions and sympathize

After delivering bad news, it is very important to allow patients to express their emotions. Remain silent at first, then offer words of reassurance. Never tell patients anything that is not factually correct, do not give them false hope.

> **Useful phrases**   I understand this is very upsetting news. Our best doctors will work with you to help you get better.

Step 6 : Strategy and summary

Bad news can be shocking, and sometimes it can be hard for patients to focus. After you explain the treatment strategy to the patient, it is important that you use the teach-back method and have the patient summarize, in their own words, what was said.

> **Useful phrases**   It's very important that you understand what we talked about here today, so I would like for you to summarize what was said in your own words.

10

Breaking bad news

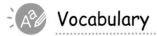 **Vocabulary**

Below is a list of key vocabulary for this chapter. Translate each word or phrase into your native language.

1. adversely _____

2. protocol _____

3. be subject to _____

4. efficacy _____

5. perspective _____

6. elicit _____

7. disclose _____

8. distressing _____

9. unwarranted _____

10. precaution _____

11. intervention _____

12. confront _____

13. ease _____

14. false hope _____

15. lessen _____

16. anxiety _____

17. agenda _____

18. technical term _____

19. constraint _____

20. interruption _____

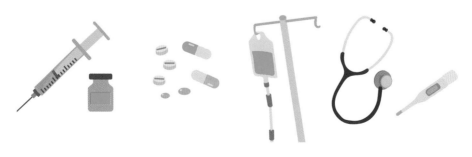

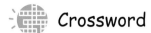

Crossword

Using the hints below, fill in the words to the puzzle.

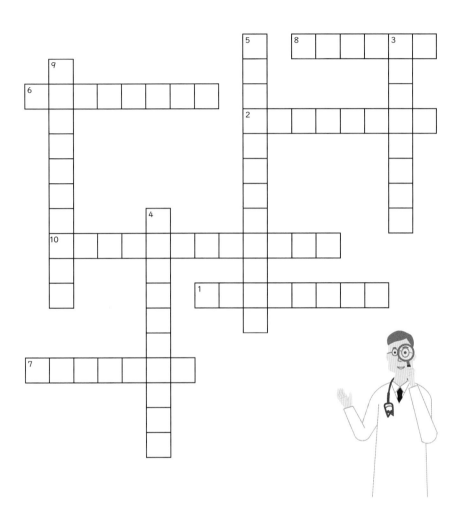

1. This is a set of procedures healthcare professionals should follow when communicating with patients.
2. This describes how well a treatment or drug achieves the desired effect.
3. This is what we do when we share confidential information.
4. This is something we do to avoid negative outcomes.
5. This is something we do to change or improve a situation.
6. This is an act of facing difficulties or to challenge someone aggressively.
7. This is a feeling of worry and restlessness.
8. This is the purpose of action or the topic one hopes to cover during a discussion.
9. This word describes a restriction or limitation.
10. This is something that bothers you or stops you when you are doing something.

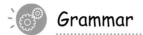

Grammar

Conjunctions

▶ **Coordinating conjunctions**

A coordinating conjunction is a "connecting word" that joins two grammatical elements of the same status: two words, two phrases, or two clauses, for example. The coordinating conjunctions in English are *for*, *and*, *nor*, *but*, *or*, *yet*, and *so*.

Ex Mary likes tea and coffee.

Ex Tom likes tea, but Jim likes coffee.

The three most common coordinating conjunctions between clauses are "and" (which normally connects two simple clauses), "but" (which connects contrasting clauses), and "so" (which connects a reason to a result).

Ex This patient was admitted today, and this patient will be admitted tomorrow.

Ex Your test results look good, but I think we should be cautious.

Ex Dr. Noguchi is in surgery at the moment, so he can't see any patients.

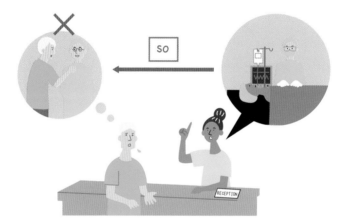

▸Subordinating conjunctions

A subordinating conjunction is used to join a sentence that adds additional information to the main clause. Typical subordinating conjunctions include *after, although, as, because, before, if, since, unless, until, when, whereas, whether,* and *while.*

In the sentence below, "because" is the subordinating conjunction. It shows the connection between the main and subordinate clauses.

`Ex` He was late for his appointment (main clause) because the train stopped (subordinate clause).

Here, "Although" is the subordinating conjunction. It shows contrast.

`Ex` Although surgery is an option (subordinate clause), I wouldn't recommend it (main clause).

A subordinate clause can come after or before a main clause. For example, you could change the first example sentence to "Because the train stopped (subordinate clause), he was late for his appointment (main clause)." When the subordinate clause comes first, it is followed by a comma.

1 Fill in the blanks with the missing conjunction. There may be more than one possible answer for each sentence.

1. Jack and Mary went to the same school (   ) they were young.

2. (   ) he was so tall, he always bumped his head.

3. You've been eating a lot of salty foods, (   ) your blood pressure is high.

4. (   ) you find the document, please let me know.

5. (   ) I exercise a lot, I keep gaining weight.

2 Read the following sentences. If the sentence uses conjunctions correctly, write "○." If it contains a mistake, write "✕." Then fix the sentence.

1. I had too much coffee, so I won't be able to sleep at night.   (   )

2. Although I'd love to attend the conference, I'm too busy to go.   (   )

3. Because I have lots of reports to write.   (   )

4. I want to become a doctor, but I'm going to go to medical school.   (   )

5. Tell me right away if you experience any pain.   (   )

📖 Reading

Read the following passage. Answer the questions in the box below.

It is important to remember that bad news is not always about telling a patient they have a fatal condition. Bad news is defined as any news that has the potential to negatively change a person's life. There are many difficult things to face that are just as frightening as death. For example, finding out that you will never be able to walk again would be very bad news. Imagine if you were told you would never be able to have children, you would lose an arm, or that you would go blind. How would that make you feel? You can be sure your patients will have similar feelings.

The most critical thing to remember about breaking bad news is what your voice and face will mean to your patients for the rest of their lives. That is because your bad news will dramatically change their lives forever. Breaking bad news should never be taken lightly. It is a very serious responsibility and should always be done with the patient's psychological well-being in mind.

Using words or phrases to help prepare patients for bad news is often called giving a warning shot. Some studies have shown that warning the patient of bad news may lessen the shock and increase the patient's ability to process the information. One example of a "warning shot" would be, "The test results are shown, and unfortunately, I do not have good news." After patients hear a sentence like this, they can know the news will be bad and mentally prepare themselves for it. It is significant for healthcare professionals to deliver bad news the proper way. When disclosing bad news, use clear and concise language. Match your words to your patients' level of understanding. Avoid using difficult medical words. Pause frequently and allow your patients to understand what you are saying. Frequently checking patients' understanding helps prevent miscommunication. Avoid phrases that are too direct, sound judgmental, or may leave the patient feeling extreme hopelessness. Remember, as a healthcare professional, you have many things to offer your patients, even with the worst prognosis.

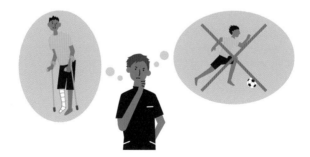

1. What is "bad news"? Please describe it in your own words.
2. Why will patients be changed by you for the rest of their lives?
3. In the text, you saw the phrase "warning shot." What is it? Please give some examples.
4. Is it difficult for you to tell someone bad news? Why?
5. Was there ever a time when you received bad news? How did you feel?

Speaking & writing

Look at the following questions. Write down your opinion in response to each question. Share your opinions with the class, in small groups, or with your teacher.

1. What emotion do you imagine a patient will feel after hearing bad news?

2. What can healthcare professionals do to help reduce the negative impact of bad news?

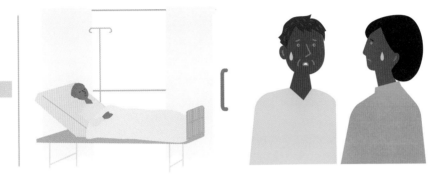

 ## What do you think?

Look at the following questions. Write down your opinion in response to each question. Share your opinions with the class, in small groups, or with your teacher.

1. What are the most important things to consider when breaking bad news?

2. How does learning how to break bad news protect you as a healthcare professional? What might happen if you are careless about conveying bad news to patients?

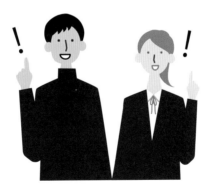

Listening practice 2

Listen to the following conversations. Write the missing words and phrases.

Track 10-2

Doctor: I am sorry to say your _____ _____ show that a tumor was found in your right breast.

Patient: Oh, no!   Am I going to die soon? _____ _____ ___ ____?

Doctor: At this stage, there are _____ _____ _____. I will go over each of those with you so that we can choose the best course of action available.

Patient: ___ ____ _____. I don't know what to say……. I want to have my family with me when you go over the treatment options. I don't think I can make the right decision on my own.

Doctor: I completely understand. This must be very difficult for you. I would like to schedule an appointment with you and your family members as soon as possible.

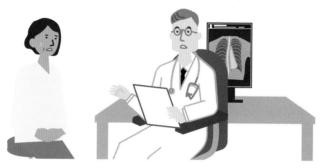

Track 10-3

Nurse: Doctor, is there anything I should be _____ of when talking to patients, especially patients who are suffering from a _____ _____?

Doctor: It's important to always show _____. Although, we can become very _____, We should not forget to show empathy. Patients with severe conditions _____ a lot of _____ _____. Your role is to offer not only _____ care but also emotional support as well. If you have to deliver bad news to a patient, always do it with empathy and _____ care.

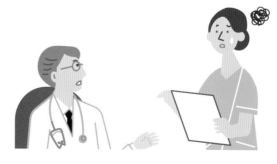

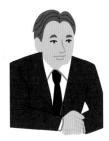

Name Hiroyuki Daida

Introduction Dr. Hiroyuki Daida is a Professor Emeritus in the Department of Cardiovascular Medicine at Juntendo University.

Comment

Interviewer: What do you have to keep in mind when treating patients?

Professor Daida: It may be simple, but I think it's important to understand and face the person as a whole human being and not just focus on the patient's illness. Because there are so many treatment options available in the current practice, it is especially important that we fully understand the patient's social background, family situation, preferences, and so on to choose an adequate therapeutic strategy for each patient.

Interviewer: Is there anything else we should keep in mind when taking a patient history, visiting patients on the ward, or breaking bad news?

Professor Daida: Because patients are often very concerned and nervous about the status of their illness, we must gently treat them and communicate in an easy-to-understand manner. That means when interacting with patients, we doctors have to be not only warm and collaborative but also objective.

Interviewer: What message do you have for healthcare students and future healthcare professionals?

Professor Daida: My message for those who have chosen to go on the medical path is this: as you firmly acquire medical skills and knowledge, do not forget to nurture your medical professional mind. No matter how advanced the medical treatment has become, the most important thing is to maintain the sensitivity to empathize with your patients. One word, one action, and one smile can help you save your patients.

11 Quality of life

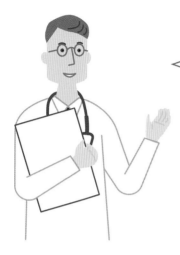

I recommend walking to the station in the morning.

"Quality of life (QOL)" refers to how good a person's life is. According to the WHO, QOL is based on how a person perceives their position in life. This is related to context, culture, and social value. It is also related to each person's goals, expectations, standards, and concerns. Finally, QOL is influenced by physical health, psychological condition, beliefs, personal relationships, and professional relationships. The primary goal of healthcare is to help patients obtain the best possible QOL.

Listening practice 1

Listen to the following track. Complete the notes below.

🔊 Track11-1

Name: _____

Age: _____

Gender: _____

Occupation: _____

Marital status: _____

Hobby: _____

Illness: _____

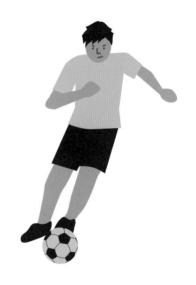

Language corner

Look at the list below. According to the WHO, these are the categories that relate to QOL.

✓ Physical health

Ex *energy, fatigue, pain, discomfort, sleep, rest*

> Useful phrases
> · How is your energy level today?

✓ Psychological

Ex *bodily image, negative feelings, positive feelings, self-esteem, thinking, learning, memory, concentration*

> Useful phrases
> · You seem down. Is there anything I can do to help?

✓ Level of independence

Ex *mobility, activities of daily living, dependence on medication and medical aids, work capacity*

> Useful phrases
> · Let's see how far you can walk on your own.

✓ Social relations

Ex *personal relationships, social support, sexual activity*

> Useful phrases
> · Is there anyone who can help?

✓ Environment

Ex *finances, freedom, safety, access to health and social care, home, learning opportunities, opportunities for recreation, community relationship, physical environment, transportation*

> Useful phrases
> · Are there places in your neighborhood where you can go to relieve stress?

✓ Spirituality/Religion/Personal beliefs

Ex *religious practice, food restrictions, culture, meaning of life*

> Useful phrases
> · Do you have a religion?
> · Would you like to have a priest or spiritual guide here for support?

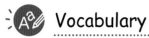 # Vocabulary

Below is a list of key vocabulary for this chapter. Translate each word or phrase into your native language.

1. quality of life _____

2. according to _____

3. context _____

4. social value _____

5. standards _____

6. concern 動 _____

7. category _____

8. physical _____

9. relationship _____

10. subjective _____

11. occupation _____

12. fatigue _____

13. palliative care _____

14. self-esteem _____

15. concentration _____

16. mobility _____

17. independence _____

18. capacity _____

19. financial _____

20. spirituality _____

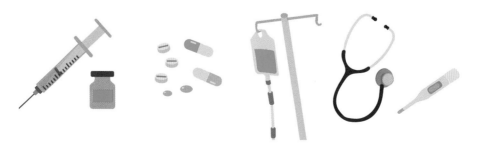

Matching
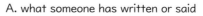

Write the letter corresponding to the description on the right.

1. quality of life _____

2. according to _____

3. context _____

4. social value _____

5. standards _____

6. concern _____

7. category _____

8. physical _____

9. relationship _____

10. subjective _____

11. occupation _____

12. fatigue _____

13. palliative care _____

14. self-esteem _____

15. concentration _____

16. mobility _____

17. independence _____

18. capacity _____

19. financial _____

20. spirituality _____

A. what someone has written or said

B. the maximum something can have or hold

C. the group something belongs to

D. deep mental focus, close gathering

E. another word for worries

F. setting, environment for words, events, and ideas

G. a medical care to optimize QOL and reduce suffering among people with serious or terminal illness

H. done under one's own control

I. the feeling of being tired

J. related to money

K. the ability to move

L. one's job

M. can be touched, seen, heard, smelled, or tasted

N. measure of how good every day is

O. connection between things or people

P. one's own pride

Q. something a group of people treasure

R. one's religious belief

S. ideas to measure quality or what is normal

T. based on personal feelings and opinions

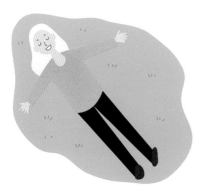

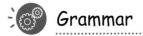 Grammar

Prepositions

A preposition is a word or a group of words used in front of a noun or a pronoun to show time, direction, or location, among other information.

▶ Simple prepositions

A simple preposition is a short word that shows a relationship with a noun or pronouns. It can also help connect parts of a sentence. Simple prepositions are usually prepositions of time, direction, or location.

Prepositions of time

These prepositions show the timing of something in relation to a noun or pronoun. Examples of prepositions of time include *after*, *before*, *at*, *on*, *in*, *during*, *since*, and *until*.

Ex **After** the operation, the doctor talked with the patient's family.

Ex My self-esteem and concentration have improved **since** February.

Prepositions of direction

Some prepositions indicate where something moves in relation to a noun or pronoun. *Across*, *along*, *around*, *down*, *from*, *into*, *off*, *over*, *through*, *to*, *toward*, and *up* are all examples of prepositions of direction.

Ex I recommend walking **to** the station in the morning.

Ex The needle injects the medication directly **into** the bloodstream.

Prepositions of place

These prepositions show where something is in relation to a noun or pronoun. Examples of place prepositions include *above*, *at*, *behind*, *below*, *beneath*, *between*, *in*, *near*, *on*, *outside*, *over*, *under*, *upon*, and *within*.

Ex Could you lift your arms **above** your head?

Ex The optimal temperature level is **between** these two values.

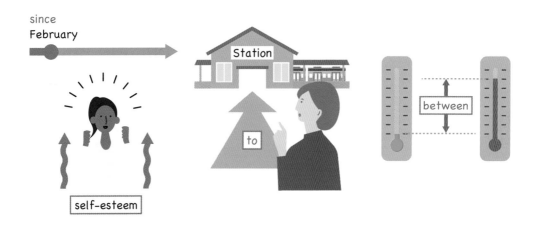

▸ **Compound prepositions**

A compound preposition, which is made up of a preposition and another word, usually comes as a set. Here are some examples: *according to, ahead of, along with, apart from, compared to, because of, except for, from above, from behind, from between, inside of, instead of, out of.*

🔑 Key Points

The key difference between prepositions and conjunctions is that prepositions tell you about a noun in terms of direction, place, or time, for example. A conjunction tells you the relationship between ideas.

Ex There are patients in the waiting room.

The preposition "in" tells you about "patients" in terms of place (the waiting room).

Ex You need rest, so you should stay home.

The conjunction "so" tells you the relationship between "You need rest" and "You should stay home" (reason and result).

---

1 Fill in the blank with a suitable preposition. There may be more than one possible answer for each sentence.

1. Please take the medication _____ eating.

2. I recommend taking walks _____ your neighborhood to stay fit.

3. _____ the exit, there's a bathroom.

4. I got a call _____ a worried patient yesterday morning.

5. Do you normally have a snack _____ bedtime?

2 Write sentences using a preposition of place or direction for each of the following verb tenses.

1. Present continuous   Ex I am walking **to** the station now.

2. Present perfect   Ex I haven't been abroad **since** high school.

3. Interrogative   Ex Can you grab the chart **on** the table?

4. Imperative   Ex Take one dose **after** breakfast.

5. Past perfect   Ex The patient had completed all of her tests **before** her reexamination.

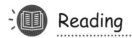

Read the following passage. Answer the questions in the box below.

Each day, millions of healthcare workers around the world are doing their best to help people overcome injury and illness. Hospital staff can become very busy. In big, crowded hospitals, healthcare professionals can sometimes care for hundreds of people a day. At worst, the hospital might resemble a place for simply fixing people. The patient comes in for exams and treatment. The patient is sent back out again. The next patient comes, and the processes repeats itself.

Over time the human side of the patient might be overlooked. The important thing to remember is that patients are not just things to fix. They have emotions. They have families and careers. They have hopes and dreams. They have a sense of pride. They want to be autonomous. They want the support of friends and the community. They want to be able to speak to their gods or understand the nature of their own existence. When healthcare professionals treat patients, they must consider not only their physical needs but also their psychological needs. They must consider how treatment will affect patients' quality of life (QOL).

Imagine that you are in a hospital right now, taking care of a patient who is in pain. Your first goal might be to help the patient by reducing his pain as much as possible. There is a drug that will help, but it will make the patient very sleepy. It will also make it difficult for him to think clearly and communicate with others. You know that your patient is a person who wants to show others that he is strong and capable. He has told you that he would rather have a clear mind than less pain. For him, a pain-free life without the ability to think clearly and speak clearly would be a poor QOL. How would you handle the situation?

It is always important to consider patients' desires to help them maintain the type of QOL they want for themselves. Healthcare professionals should find a balance between their goal to heal and keeping the best QOL. In other words, future healthcare professionals should view their patients as more than machines that need to be fixed. They should see them as a whole human. When choosing the best treatment, healthcare workers should think about how that treatment will affect the patients' QOL.

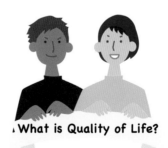

What is Quality of Life?

1. Please explain the meaning of the phrase "patients are more than machines that need to be fixed".
2. According to the article, why might the hospital feel like a place of fixing people?
3. What would you do if you were in charge of taking care of the patient that was mentioned in the article?

Speaking & writing

Look at the following questions. Write down your opinion in response to each question. Share your opinions with the class, in small groups, or with your teacher.

1. Describe your day. Think of things you routinely do every day.

2. Imagine how you would feel if you were forced to change your routine because of illness.

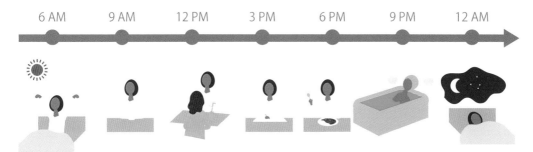

 # What do you think?

Look at the following questions. Write down your opinion in response to each question. Share your opinions with the class, in small groups, or with your teacher.

1. Some countries consider the right to end one's own life a part of basic human rights. How do you feel about that?

2. What does death mean for you?

Listening practice 2

Listen to the following tracks. Complete the notes below.

🔊 Track 11-2

Physical health: _____

Psychological state: _____

Level of independence: _____

Social relations: _____

Environment: _____

Spirituality: _____

🔊 Track 11-3

Physical health: _____

Psychological state: _____

Level of independence: _____

Social relations: _____

Environment: _____

Spirituality: _____

🔊 Track 11-4

Physical health: _____

Psychological state: _____

Level of independence: _____

Social relations: _____

Environment: _____

Spirituality: _____

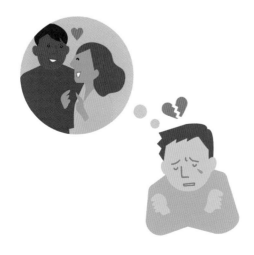

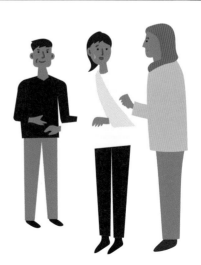

Professional profiles

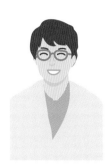

Name Mari Saito

Introduction Dr. Mari Saito is a palliative care specialist with over 20 years of experience caring for terminally ill patients.

Comment My specialty is palliative care. One of the main goals of healthcare professionals working in palliative care is to help patients feel more comfortable by reducing their pain. However, due to the nature of the disease, it is sometimes impossible to eliminate pain completely. In these cases, the goal is to reduce pain as much as possible and maintain quality of life (QOL). However, QOL is subjective. It means something different to each person. That is why healthcare professionals must always consider the balance between treatment goals and the desires of their patients, which we learn by talking with them and their families.

I love studying English because it teaches me new ways to express myself. As I learn how to communicate with English, I also learn how to use words more effectively. Sometimes it's difficult for me to say some things in English and I have to use simpler language to do it. English also makes me aware of body language and other nonverbal types of communication. Through studying English, I learn how to better listen to and communicate with my patients.

 # Homework

. . . .

1 Based on the WHO's six measures of QOL, write about your own QOL.

2 Interview someone and assess his or her QOL based on the six categories established by the WHO. Use the information you have gathered to write a brief report on the person you have interviewed.

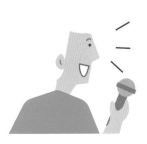
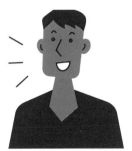

Chapter 12 Aging

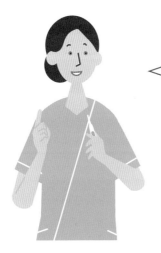

> Getting old is a part of life.

"Do not scold the young, for you were once one of them. Do not scorn the old, for you will be one of them." As this proverb suggests, aging is an inevitable part of human life. Japan, with its declining birth rate and long life expectancies, is becoming a "super-aging society" and setting an example of older adult care for other countries. Communication is a vital part of that process. In this chapter, we will discuss how to communicate with older adult patients in an empathetic and caring way.

Listening practice 1

Listen to the following track. Choose the right word or phrase for each sentence.

🔊 Track 12-1

1. Sunnydale is for (older adults / children).
2. The staff at Sunnydale must always (entertain / respect) the patients.
3. The top concern is patients' (defense / dignity).
4. According the speaker, the (patients' / staff's) needs are the most important.

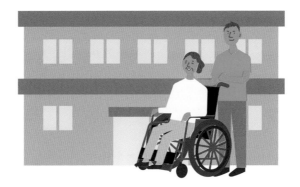

Listening practice 2

Listen to the following conversation between a nurse and a care worker (CW). Write the missing words and phrases.

🔊 Track 12-2

Nurse: Hello!   Nice to meet you. One of our patients will be checking into the care home tomorrow, _____ _____ his family. I wanted to talk with you about his health status.

CW: Sure. I'm the care manager in charge of the patient. Let me take some notes so that I don't miss any important information. First, can you tell me ___ _____ ____ about the patient?

Nurse: He is 86 years old and _____ _____ Alzheimer's disease. While he is not bedridden, he is becoming _____. He has limited mobility and needs a wheelchair to get around. At home, he usually uses a walking aid.

CW: OK. How about his sanitary _____?

Nurse: He bathes with the help of a care worker. He needs a little help going to the bathroom. He uses incontinence pads during the night.

CW: What about his mental capacity?

Nurse: ____ _____ _____ _____. He is normally fine—he can have conversations, but he occasionally forgets where he is and feels _____ sometimes. According to his family, when he has a tough time, he often remembers his hometown near the sea. It seems as if he is trying to get back to that place in his mind. _____ _____ _____, we show him pictures from his childhood to _____ _____ _____.

CW: What else should we know?

Nurse: He used to be a businessperson, and he is very happy when he talks about his travels _____.

CW: I'll remember that! Thanks for all the information.

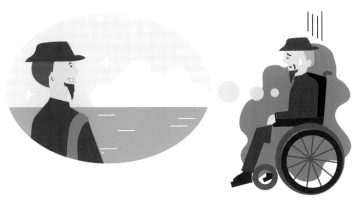

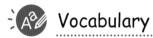 Vocabulary

Below is a list of key vocabulary for this chapter. Translate each word or phrase into your native language.

1. respect _____

2. stimulation _____

3. bedridden _____

4. aid _____

5. memory _____

6. dementia _____

7. proactive _____

8. nursing home _____

9. older adult _____

10. humiliate _____

11. humanity _____

12. patience _____

13. dignity _____

14. impairment _____

15. routine _____

16. fragile _____

17. frail _____

18. confusion _____

19. incontinence _____

20. restricted _____

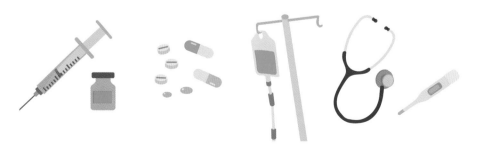

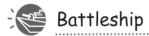 # Battleship

1. You have four ships of varying lengths. Place your ships on the map. Ships can be placed vertically and horizontally.
2. Take turns trying to find your partner's ships by stating coordinates, one from the left and one from the top (**Ex** Respect/Humanity). When saying the coordinates, be sure to read the words out loud.
3. For example, if your submarine is at 10-A (Humiliate/Humanity) and 10-B (Humiliate/Patience), and your partner calls out, "Is there something at Humiliate and Humanity?", your partner will get a point because he or she will have found part of your ship.
4. The winner is the one who finds all of his or her partner's ships first or has the most points.

Battleship					Cruiser				
Carrier						Submarine			

My Ships		A Humanity	B Patience	C Dignity	D Impairment	E Routine	F Fragile	G Frail	H Confusion	I Incontinence	J Restricted
1	Respect										
2	Stimulation										
3	Bedridden										
4	Aid										
5	Memory										
6	Dementia										
7	Proactive										
8	Nursing home										
9	Older adult										
10	Humiliate										

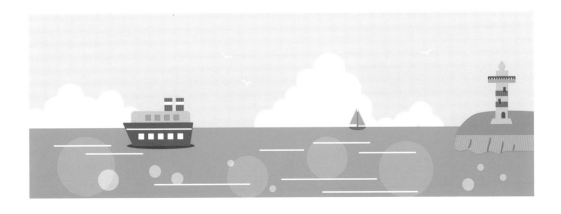

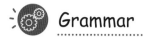 **Grammar**

Infinitives/Gerunds

▸ Infinitives

An infinitive (also called a "to-infinitive") is generally the base form of a verb with "to" in front of it.

Ex **to sit, to walk, to live**

Infinitives serve different purposes in sentences. They can be the subject of the sentence or additional information (as an abjective or an adverb). However, a sentence with an infinitive as its subject often sounds formal and sometimes stiff.

Ex I see the doctor every week **to undergo** treatment.

Ex **To get** to the radiology department, go to the third floor./Go to the third floor **to get** to the radiology department. (In the examples, "to undergo…" and "to get…" mark the beginning of additional information.)

Ex **To visit** Norway is my dream. (This is a little stiff.)

▸ Gerunds

A gerund is a verbal noun: a form of a verb ending in **-ing** that functions as a noun. A gerund can be the subject or object of a sentence.

Ex **Running** makes me tired.

Ex I hate **taking** powdered medicine.

▸ Deciding between infinitives and gerunds

When to use infinitives

(1) If you're using a verb after an adjective, you often use the infinitive.

　　Ex It's hard **to turn** my head to the right.

(2) The infinitive is the best choice for indicating purpose.

　　Ex The patient's family came to me **to get** a second opinion on his dementia.

When to use gerunds

(1) Gerunds are generally the best choice after a preposition.

　　Ex The team gave the patient anesthesia before **beginning** the surgery.

(2) Gerunds tend to be the best for replacing a subject or object.

　　Ex **Getting** old is a part of life.

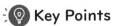 Key Points

Some verbs have different meanings in the infinitive and gerund forms. Examples include remember, forget, and stop.

The important differences are:

(1) The infinitive is for things that have not happened yet, while the gerund is for things that have already happened; and

(2) The infinitive shows purpose

Remember to lock the door.	I remember locking the door.
The action (to lock the door) has not happened yet. The person is telling someone to do that action in the future.	The action (locking) has already happened, and the person remembers that event.

1 Fill in the blanks. Write the appropriate form of the verb (infinitive or gerund).

1. After _____ (complete) the treatment, the patient felt much better.

2. I take several medications _____ (control) my blood pressure.

3. The doctor recommended _____ (avoid) fatty foods.

2 Look at the sentences below. Find the mistakes and correct them.

1. Feel free to discussing this question with your classmates if you think it's necessary.

2. Before deciding to study medicine, I thought about going abroad learning English.

3. Going upstairs is hard to do because I run out of breath when do physical activity.

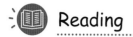 **Reading**

Read the following passage. Answer the questions in the box below.

"Humanitude" is French for "humanity." It is a caretaking method created in 1979 by Gineste Eve and Rosette Marescotti, two French gymnastic teachers. Humanitude is a way of caring for older adult patients that is based on a philosophy of showing respect for their dignity.

As we have seen in previous chapters, healthcare professionals should treat all patients as fellow human beings in need of care. Even when patients with dementia, for example, are unable to respond to their caregivers, the healthcare professionals need to express their concern for their patients' well-being.

The Humanitude method requires caregivers to communicate through four key elements: seeing, talking, touching, and being with patients. These four elements allow caregivers to connect with their patients on an emotional level. This method is also very useful for preventing agitation, anger, and inactivity in patients. Humanitude allows caregivers to respond flexibly to a variety of situations.

The five steps of Humanitude are as follows.

1) Prepare yourself to meet the patient. Treat the patient as your friend. By doing so, you help the patient's brain prepare itself to meet people and accept visitors.

2) Prepare yourself to care for the patient. Instead of trying to save time by offering care right away, build a relationship through small talk. Then suggest the type of care that you intend to offer (bathing, medication, etc.) so that the patient can accept it more autonomously.

3) Through seeing, talking, and touching, communicate the feeling that you care for the patient.

4) Create emotional attachment. Even senile patients retain memories of kindness and good impressions. Make sure to establish rapport.

5) Promise to see the patient again. Tell the patient that you will come back. The patient will thus look forward to seeing you which will facilitate the next meeting.

The Humanitude method is now being used in many countries, including Japan. It helps caregivers build empathetic connections with patients and makes emotion an important part of a new standard in caretaking.

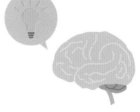

---

1. What is the basic principle of the Humanitude method?

2. When and by whom was the method created?

3. What are the four elements of Humanitude?

4. What are the five steps of the Humanitude method?

Speaking & writing

Think about someone you are close to that is an older adult.

1. Imagine what that person was like when they were younger. How do you imagine that person has changed over the years?
2. What can you do to help improve that person's life?

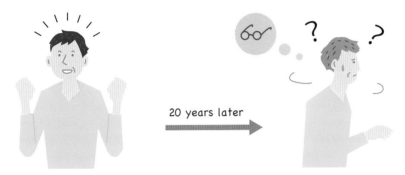

20 years later

 ## What do you think?

Look at the following questions. Write down your opinion in response to each question. Share your opinions with the class, in small groups, or with your teacher.

1. What are some memorable experiences you have had with an older adult?
2. What can people do to make living environments better for older adults?
3. In what way could technology be useful in older adult care? Do you think AI and other technologies can change older adult care?

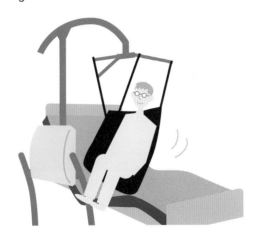

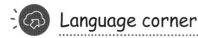 **Language corner**

Caring for older adults is an important part of healthcare. Below are some idiomatic expressions, words, and sentences you can use when caring for older adults.

✅ Idiomatic expressions related to age

- **Golden years** : "Marc is 70. He is in his golden years."
- **Feel one's age** : "Climbing the stairs is hard for her. She's starting to feel her age."
- **Young at heart** : "They are in their 80s and energetic. They are young at heart."
- **To be pushing an age** : "Although he looks young, he must be pushing 60."

✅ Expressions related to healthcare

- **Dementia** : "Lately, he seems confused. He may be suffering from dementia."
- **Regimen** : "She must take a daily regimen of medications to maintain her health."
- **Home care** : "He doesn't want to go to a hospice, so he will receive home care instead."
- **Nursing home** : "Her children can't care for her. They placed her in a nursing home."

✅ Encouraging words

- You are doing great. Let's try one more time.
- You look very cheerful today.
- You are almost done with dinner, just one more bite.
- Well done.

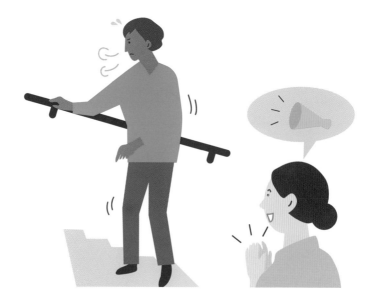

Origin of medical gloves

Read the following passage. Answer the questions in the box below.

Today, gloves are one of the most common medical supplies found in hospitals. They are essential because they can prevent the spread of infection to patients and doctors during surgery and other treatments. Although they are quite ordinary, medical gloves have an interesting origin story, which came from a warm-hearted coincidence.

The rubber gloves worn during surgery were invented in 1890 by William Stewart Halstead of Johns Hopkins University, who is known as the "Father of the Resident System." The invention was for his girlfriend Caroline, who was a nurse. At that time, all surgical operations were performed with bare hands. The surgeons and surgical assistants had to immerse their hands in a powerful antiseptic solution to sanitize them. Dr. Halstead was wondering if there was a way for Caroline, whose skin was weak, to avoid getting rough hands and skin damage from using the antiseptic solution. So, he came up with the idea of rubber gloves! He asked the Goodyear Rubber Co., which was located next to the hospital, to make two pairs of thin rubber gloves to protect her hands. Soon after, surgeons found out about Caroline's gloves and news spread across the world. Goodyear was flooded with orders to make more.

Dr. Halstead realized a few years later that wearing gloves could not only protect a surgeon's skin but also prevent infectious diseases. As a preventive measure for the spread of bacteria, wearing gloves was more potent than soaking one's hands in a disinfectant solution. Gloves are now an indispensable part of medicine.

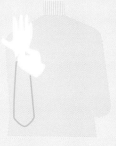

1. What was Dr. Halstead's initial purpose for making surgical gloves?
2. Before gloves were invented, what method had been used to protect the medical staff and patients from infection?
3. If you could invent anything for the medical field, real or imagined, what would you invent and why?
4. What is your overall thought about the reading?

13 Diversity

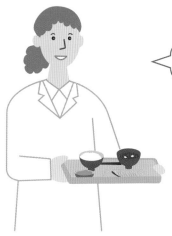

> Could you tell me about your culture?

If you travel abroad and fall sick, you may feel uneasy, especially if you do not understand the spoken language. Most people can understand the importance of good communication and feeling comfortable in a foreign environment, especially in the medical setting. It is important for all healthcare professionals to bridge cultural and linguistic gaps when providing appropriate medical care at hospitals. Let's take a closer look at what is needed to improve cultural competence in healthcare.

🎧 Listening practice 1

Listen to the following conversation between a receptionist and a patient. Complete the notes below.

🔊 Track13-1

Name: _____

Appointment time: _____

Type of insurance: _____

Symptom: _____

Department: _____

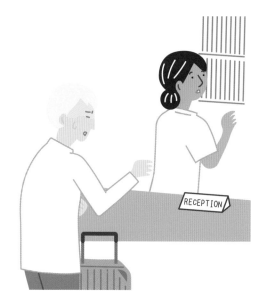

Listening practice 2

Listen to the following conversation between a receptionist and a patient. Write the missing words and phrases.

🔊 Track 13-2

Receptionist: Here is a _____ _____ for you to fill out.

Please write your full name here.

Please write your home address and contact information.

Now, in this box, please put your _____ ____ _____.

Write the year first, _____ _____ the month, and then write the day here in the last space.

Would you like me to _____ _____ this form _____ your _____?

Patient: Yes, please.

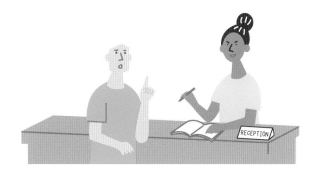

🔊 Track 13-3

Receptionist: Today's fee is _____ yen.

Patient: Here you go.

Receptionist: Although you have to pay the total fee upfront, you should be able to get a _____ _____ your _____ _____.

Patient: Oh, OK.

Receptionist: These are the documents for the _____ _____.

Patient: Thanks. So, I should send them to the _____ company?

Receptionist: Yes, that's right.

Patient: Thank you very much for your help.

Receptionist: You're welcome. _____ _____ _____.

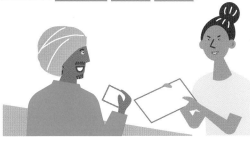

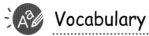 # Vocabulary

Below is a list of key vocabulary for this chapter. Translate each word or phrase into your native language.

1. awareness _____

2. diversity _____

3. religious _____

4. restriction _____

5. dietary _____

6. culture _____

7. end-of-life _____

8. Judaism _____

9. Islam _____

10. Hinduism _____

11. Buddhism _____

12. cultural competence _____

13. folk therapy _____

14. ethnicity _____

15. preventive medicine _____

16. stereotype _____

17. values _____

18. intercultural communication _____

19. socioeconomic status _____

20. sexual orientation _____

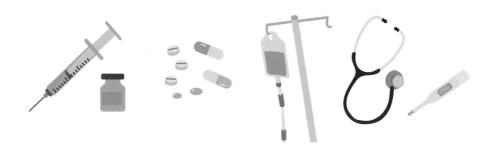

Matching

Write the letter corresponding to the description on the right.

1. awareness _____
2. diversity _____
3. religious _____
4. restriction _____
5. dietary _____
6. culture _____
7. end-of-life _____
8. Judaism _____
9. Islam _____
10. Hinduism _____
11. Buddhism _____
12. cultural competence _____
13. folk therapy _____
14. ethnicity _____
15. preventive medicine _____
16. stereotype _____
17. values _____
18. intercultural communication _____
19. socioeconomic status _____
20. sexual orientation _____

A. something that limits something else
B. medical techniques and treatments intended to prevent disease before it happens
C. a fixed image that many people have of a particular type of person
D. an ability to interact effectively with people of different cultures
E. knowing about the existence of something
F. related to someone's death and the time just before it
G. how one judges what is important in life and their standards of behavior
H. one's natural preference for a particular gender as a sex partner
I. related to the food one regularly eats
J. a religion based on the teachings of Siddhartha Gautama
K. the religion of the Jewish people
L. the social standing or class of an individual or group based on wealth or position
M. a range of people of things from many different cultural and ethnic backgrounds
N. the fact of belonging to a particular nation or people
O. the religion practiced by Muslims
P. traditional treatments that have not been prescribed by a doctor
Q. the art and actions shared by a group of people
R. the most common religion in India.
S. communication across nationalities and races
T. the relation to or belief in a religion

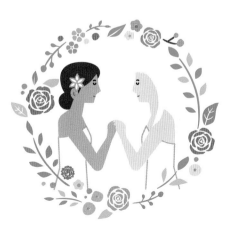

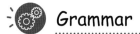

Grammar

Auxiliary verbs

▸ Should

Use **should** when you want to give a recommendation, ask a question about what to do, or say something is expected.

Ex You **should** try to avoid stereotypes.

Ex **Should** I take this after lunch?

Ex The doctor **should** be free next Friday. (= I expect the doctor to be free.)

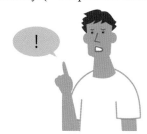

▸ Could

Use **could** to express possibility, make a polite request, or as the past tense of can.

Ex We **could** eat out.

Ex **Could** you tell me about your culture?

Ex I **could** run without pain yesterday.

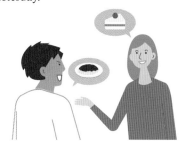

▸ Would

Use **would** to make a polite request or invitation, describe hypothetical situations, or express a past habit.

Ex **Would** you hand me his chart?

Ex If I were you, I **would** stop smoking.

Ex My mom **would** often take a nap after lunch. (= She did this regularly.)

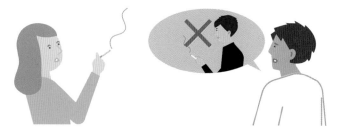

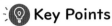

Key Points

- **Should** is weaker than **must** or **have to.**
  - **Ex** You should go there. (= You still have a choice not to go.)
    You must/have to go there. (= You have no alternative but to go.)
- Both **could** and **would** can be used for polite requests. In that usage, **could** is more common and **would** is more formal.
- **Would** is often used in sentences with **if** to describe hypothetical (imagined) situations that have a lower probability of occurring.

Fill in the blanks with the missing words. Choose from these auxiliary verbs.

> should / could / would

1. I don't think you _____ keep taking that medication.

2. If you had the chance to go back to school, _____ you study medicine again?

3. His dietary restrictions _____ have a negative effect on the treatment's effectiveness. We just don't know at this point.

4. Based on your symptoms, I think you _____ have the flu.

5. Doctors _____ always have an awareness of cultural differences.

6. _____ you be able to come in for another appointment next week?

7. I'm optimistic about this treatment. Due to her young age, the patient _____ respond well.

8. My mom _____ tell me to get a lot of sleep whenever I got sick as a child.

9. I _____ lift heavy things before I injured my back.

10. _____ I be worried about my test results?

📖 Reading

Read the following passage. Answer the questions in the box below.

There is a growing need for cultural competence in medical settings in Japan. Bridging cultural and linguistic gaps when providing appropriate medical care at hospitals is an important issue for all healthcare professionals. In spite of this, cultural competence in healthcare has received little attention in recent years.

Cultural awareness is not unique. We often face and must get along with people from different cultures. Everyone has their own unique culture. There are even certain cultures among medical professionals, such as the cultures associated with being a nurse or surgeon. In spite of this, many Japanese healthcare professionals are not accustomed to communicating with and caring for international patients.

One of the reasons why Japanese medical professionals are not used to communicating with international patients is that many Japanese have not been exposed to cultural behavior that is not Japanese. For example, there are many religions in the world: Christianity, Buddhism, Hindu, Islam, Judaism, and so on. Each one has a set of behaviors and customs. Some religions require dietary restrictions. Other religions require men and women to be treated differently. Female adherents of some religions are more comfortable communicating with medical professionals of the same sex. Because of their lack of experience with these situations, many Japanese people cannot imagine behavior based on specific religious beliefs.

Cultural diversity in medical settings also includes things like values, expression of pain, pregnancy and birth, end-of-life (palliative) care, and health beliefs and practices. For example, research done in various countries showed two trends. First, people with low socioeconomic status are less likely to be concerned about preventive medicine. Second, Asians tend to be more stoic and not express pain. Of course, further research is required to confirm these trends. However, they tell us valuable information about cultural differences and how they affect healthcare. Some ethnic folk remedies can be unscientific but remain an important part of healthcare for certain populations.

Stereotypes hinder mutual understanding. We need to avoid them while remaining aware of the fact that cultural differences are important for developing cultural competence in medical settings. In the future, programs that foster cultural competence could be included in medical, nursing, co-medical, and health sciences education. In order to better understand international patients, trying to put ourselves in their shoes can be the first step toward mutual understanding.

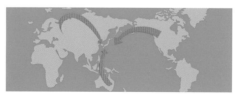

1. Explain the meaning of the word "cultural competence" in your own words.
2. According to the article, why should we avoid stereotypes?
3. If you were a patient in another country, what do you think your concerns would be?
4. In general, what stereotypes do you think you have?

Speaking & writing

Look at the following questions. Write down your opinion in response to each question. Share your opinions with the class, in small groups, or with your teacher.

1. Why is it important to think about diversity in healthcare?
2. Do you think the society you live in is diverse? Why or why not?
3. Do you want your town to be more diverse? Why or why not?

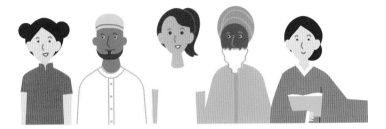

 ## What do you think?

Look at the following questions. Write down your opinion in response to each question. Share your opinions with the class, in small groups, or with your teacher.

1. How can you develop cultural competence in healthcare? Choose an example and explain it in your own words.
2. What do you think is needed to make patients feel comfortable? Please answer from the viewpoint of verbal communication and nonverbal communication.
3. What are the challenges and benefits of a more diverse hospital?

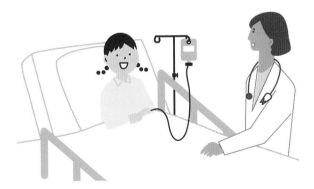

Language corner

Look at the list below. These are the list of questions you can use to treat international patients.

✅ Values

· What are the views on gender roles in your country?
· Is your country a collectivist society or an individualistic society?
· How does society view elders in your country?
· What is the social attitude towards sex in your society?
· How does your society view drinking and doing drugs.
· How does your society view mental illness?

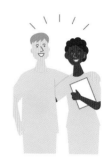

✅ Expression of pain

· In your country, how does one typically express pain?
  – Is it shameful to show pain?
  – Are there any expectations based on gender?
· How do people in your country typically feel about taking medication?

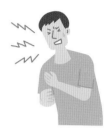

✅ Pregnancy and birth

· Does your country regularly carry out pregnancy screening?
· Is a family member expected to be present at birth in your society?
· Are there any customs or rituals associated with childbirth?

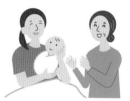

✅ End-of-life (palliative) care

· Do you want to be told about life how long you have to live?
· Do you want the doctor to tell a family member how long you have to live?
· What are your beliefs about life after death?

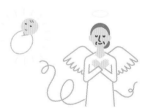

✅ Health beliefs and practices

· What are your views on organ transplants?
· Do you want to make your own healthcare decisions?
· Are there any popular folk remedies specific to your culture?
· In your culture or country, is there a stigma toward a particular disease?

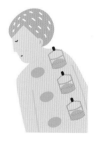

Dr. Gautam Deshpande

Read the following passage. Answer the questions written in the box below.

Dr. Gautam Deshpande is a US embassy doctor in Japan and also a general practitioner at St. Luke's International Hospital and Juntendo University Hospital.

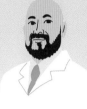

I am an Indian-American, born in a neighborhood with lots of cultural diversity. It was a great way to grow up, seeing the world from so many different perspectives. Before going to medical school, I went to college and studied human evolution while doing my pre-medical requirements. I became very interested in medical anthropology. Before medical school, I spent a year in Japan teaching medical English, which was a great experience that taught me a lot about teaching.

When I was a child, I often visited India. It was a very formative experience which left a strong impression on me that made me choose a career that allowed me to help people in need.

Listening carefully to the patient's story is the only way to really understand their illness. I try to think of every patient—no matter how scared or angry they are—as my mother, father, sister, brother, or child; it keeps my emotional energy positive.

Being a doctor, you will always be very busy and there will be a lot of pressure. We often hold patients' lives in our hands. Remain humble and never stop learning from your patients, your peers, and your community.

1. Why did he decide to become a doctor?
2. In his childhood, what kind of situation was he brought up in?
3. Does he have any difficulties being a doctor? If so, what are they?
4. What is his advice for future doctors?
5. What does the phrase "remain humble" mean to you?

13

Diversity

14 Disaster medicine

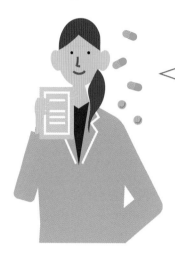

> We will let you know when it's OK to go home.

According to the United Nations Office for Disaster Risk Reduction (UNDRR), a disaster is something that causes society or a community to stop working. It is a dangerous event that causes human, material, economic, or environmental loss or damage. Recently, disasters have been increasing worldwide. There are natural disasters, such as typhoons and earthquakes. There are also man-made disasters, such as war or environmental contamination. Disaster medicine combines emergency medicine and disaster management. The goal is to treat patients who have suffered from a disaster.

💡 Key Points

Types of disasters :

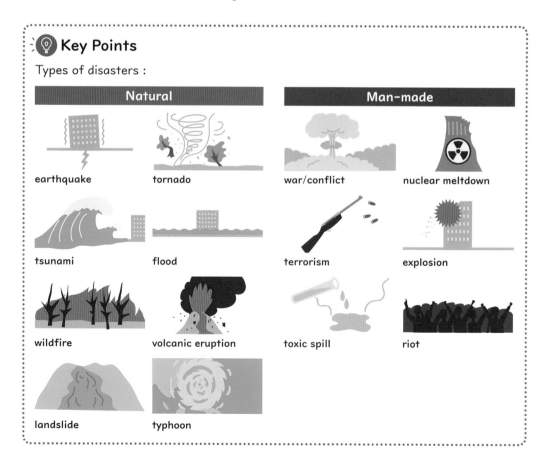

Natural		Man-made	
earthquake	tornado	war/conflict	nuclear meltdown
tsunami	flood	terrorism	explosion
wildfire	volcanic eruption	toxic spill	riot
landslide	typhoon		

Listening practice 1

Listen to the following lecture and discussion. Answer the following questions.

◀)) Track 14-1

1. Why did the class laugh?
2. According to The United Nations Office for Disaster Risk Reduction, what does the word disaster mean?
3. What are the two types of disasters mentioned by the professor, and what are some examples of each?
4. What is the difference between a hurricane, typhoon, and cyclone?
5. What do you suppose the professor meant by "That is a good question"?

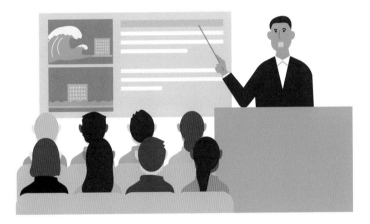

 ## Listening practice 2

Listen to the following descriptions. What disaster is the narrator talking about in each one? Write your answers below.

◀)) Track 14-2

1. _____
2. _____
3. _____
4. _____
5. _____

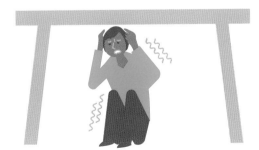

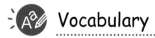 # Vocabulary

Below is a list of key vocabulary for this chapter. Translate each word or phrase into your native language.

1. tornado _____

2. flood _____

3. wildfire _____

4. volcanic eruption _____

5. landslide _____

6. hurricane _____

7. conflict _____

8. nuclear meltdown _____

9. terrorism _____

10. explosion _____

11. toxic spill _____

12. riot _____

13. triage _____

14. shelter _____

15. evacuate _____

16. higher ground _____

17. rescue _____

18. being prepared _____

19. coordinate _____

20. man-made _____

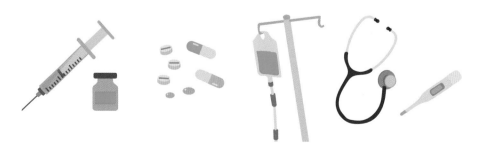

Crossword

Using the hints below, fill in the words to the puzzle.

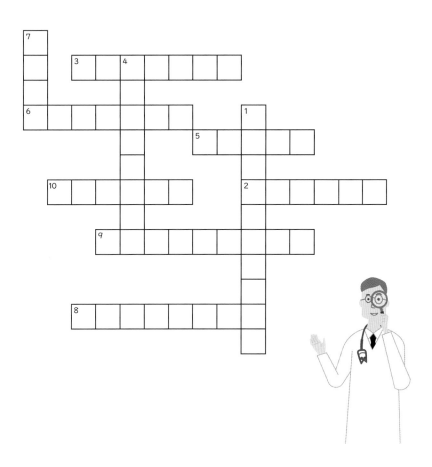

1. This word means to organize something.

2. This is what you do when you save someone.

3. This is where you go when you lose your home to disaster.

4. This is what you do when you run away for safety.

5. This happens sometimes when there is too much rain.

6. This is a violent, destructive rotating wind accompanied by a funnel-shaped cloud.

7. This is what happens when people violently protest.

8. This is another word for war.

9. This is the unlawful use of violence and intimidation for political aims.

10. This is the process of sorting patients based on the severity of their condition.

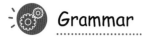 Grammar

Causative verbs

As the name suggests, "causative" verbs show that someone or something caused something to happen. In English, the most common causative verbs are *have, get, make, let,* and *help.* They have slightly different meanings, but their usage patterns are all the same—except for one.

▶ Have

There are a few ways to use "**have**," which means that someone does something for you because you pay or ask them to do it. In many cases, that "something" is part of the person's responsibility.

Ex Let's **have** the team members collaborate on the care plan.

Ex I'll **have** the patient go down to the first floor for some tests.

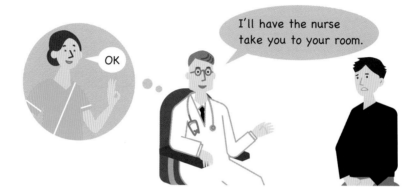

▶ Get

To "**get**" someone to do something means that you persuade them to do something. Whereas "have" means just paying or asking a person to do something, "get" is less neutral; it either involves some persuasion, isn't part of the person's normal responsibility, or is simply less formal than "have." **This is the one causative verb with a different usage pattern**: **get** + person + **to** + main verb.

Ex I **got** Dr. Egawa **to** take my patients in the afternoon. (It is not normally Dr. Egawa's job to take the speaker's patients.)

Ex Sally's father **got** her **to** come in for an appointment. (Here, Sally did not necessarily want to come in for an appointment; her father persuaded her.)

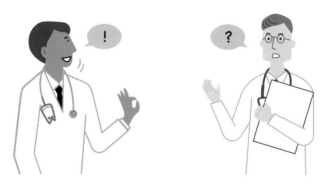

▸ Make

When you "**make**" someone do something, you force them to do it—they have no choice.

Ex My doctor **made** me stop drinking.

Ex The experience **made** me rethink my lifestyle.

▸ Let

When you "**let**" someone do something, you allow them to do it. That person wants to do it, and you give them permission.

Ex My mom **lets** me watch TV after dinner.

Ex I'll **let** you know when I'm finished.

▸ Help

The last main causative verb is "**help**." It is used to show that someone is helping someone else to do something.

Ex Social workers can **help** care teams do good work.

Ex The nursing staff **helps** some patients eat their meals.

Write your original sentences using the words and phrases given. Remember to change the causative verb to match the subject.

1. the doctor, the patient, and let

2. I, pharmacy, and had

3. the medication, patients, and make

4. the doctor, me, and got

5. the treatment, many patients, and help

📖 Reading

Read the following passage. Answer the questions in the box below.

Disaster medicine not only deals with physical health but also deals with mental health issues that can arise from a disaster. Psychiatrists and other mental healthcare workers play a big part in Disaster Medicine. They can help evaluate a group of people or a community to see how badly their mental health has been damaged after a disaster. They can support people who have been affected. Psychiatrists and psychologists can also use their experience and expertise to train staff and guide volunteer groups.

During and after a disaster, some people may need mental health support. Individuals, families, and entire communities can be affected. People can have tremendous loss as a result of man-made or natural disasters. Some people may lose their homes, lose their loved ones, be separated from their family or community, or witness violence or death. There are many things that can affect how people react. These include the following.

- type of disaster and how bad it is · past experience with disaster · how much support is available
- physical health · mental health · cultural backgrounds · age

Although most people can recover from the hardship of disaster, some people need extra help. It could be because of their age. For example children and older adults may need extra help because of their age. Some may need extra help because they have mental or physical health problems. It could also be that people need extra help because they belong to a group that is treated badly by society or they are a target of violence.

Psychological first aid (PFA) provides care and support to victims of disaster. PFA checks people's needs and worries, helps people with basic things such as food, water, and information. PFA gives people a chance to talk to someone without putting pressure on them to talk. PFA comforts people so they can feel calm and helps people connect to information, services, and support. PFA also works to protect people from more harm.

It is not necessary for PFA staff to be psychiatrists or psychologists. However, they should work with local communities to help guide and train people who volunteer to do PFA. In this way, mental healthcare professionals can support efforts made by other teams, such as nurses, medical doctors, firefighters, police, community leaders, and volunteers.

1. Why are mental healthcare professionals an important part of disaster medicine?
2. What jobs do mental healthcare professionals have in disaster medicine?
3. Why would some people need extra help after a disaster?
4. What do PFA staff provides?
5. Who can become a PFA provider?

Speaking & writing

What types of disasters has your country faced in the past?

Natural	Man-made
1.	1.
2.	2.
3.	3.
4.	4.
5.	5.

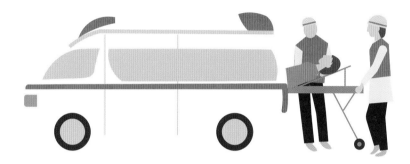

What do you think?

Look at the following questions. Write down your opinion in response to each question. Share your opinions with the class, in small groups, or with your teacher.

1. Of all the possible types of disaster, what do you think is the worst and why?
2. What are the most common disasters in your country? How do people prepare for them?
3. What is the worst disaster you have personally experienced?
4. In your opinion, what is the worst disaster in human history? Why do you think it is the worst?
5. Would you want to work in the field of disaster medicine? Why or why not?

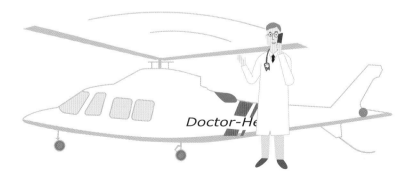

Doctor-He

14 Disaster medicine

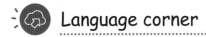

Language corner

Here are eight idiomatic expressions you can use during a disaster. Let's check each expression.

✔ Hold on for dear life

This means to hold onto something as hard as you can, usually to avoid injury.

> **Useful phrases**
> · During the flood, we held on to a tree for dear life.

✔ Out of harm's way

This means to be in a safe place, away from danger.

> **Useful phrases**
> · Because the fire only burned in the valley, the animals in the mountains were out of harm's way.

✔ Be on the safe side

This means to avoid risk.

> **Useful phrases**
> · We should turn off the gas to be on the safe side.

✔ Take cover

This means to go somewhere that shields you from danger.

> **Useful phrases**
> · During an earthquake, you should take cover under a sturdy table.

✔ At stake

This means to be in a situation where something can be lost.

> **Useful phrases**
> · The conflict has to end quickly. A lot of lives are at stake.

✔ Ride out

This means to wait for something difficult to end.

> **Useful phrases**
> · We will ride out this storm till morning.

✔ Close shave

This means a situation in which you come very close to danger.

> **Useful phrases**
> · Someone caught my arm before I fell onto the train tracks. That was a close shave!

✔ The coast is clear

This means a situation in which there is no danger present.

> **Useful phrases**
> · I checked the road ahead. There were no rioters. The coast is clear.

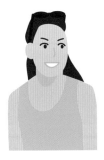

Professional profiles

Name Tomoko Kaneda

Introduction Tomoko Kaneda is a clinical psychologist based in Tokyo.

Comment I am a psychologist and I work with families who are facing psychological issues. I received my training in the United States. Studying English gave me the opportunity to learn about psychological techniques that are not being practiced in Japan. It also gave me an opportunity to meet new people from many countries and share knowledge about psychological care. I was able to apply my knowledge during the coronavirus pandemic. Because of my workplace environment, I saw many more clients who were indirectly affected by the coronavirus than those who were directly affected. I realized that my role as a healthcare professional was to offer psychological support not only to patients who had been infected but also to people who were suffering because of a loss of work or stress related to the pandemic. Due to self-restraint, schools closing, and people working from home, there was an increase in domestic problems such as violence, child abuse, and anxiety over marital relationships and childcare. My job was to help people overcome mental hardships, which can be as devastating as the disease.

 Homework

Look at the following questions. Write down your opinion for each question. Share your opinions with the class, in small groups, or with your teacher.

1. Do you know how to protect yourself when a natural disaster strikes? Discuss some common ways to protect against natural disasters.
2. In your opinion, what mental difficulties can be caused by natural disasters?
3. The important idea in disaster medicine care is expressed as "3Ts." What does "3Ts" mean? Use the internet to help you find the answer.

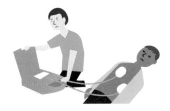

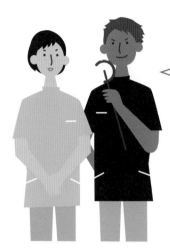

> If we work together, we will succeed.

We have examined various situations concerning healthcare and communication throughout this textbook. In the final chapter, we will discuss team care, or interprofessional care, which is healthcare given by two or more healthcare professionals. Teams include healthcare providers who have various complementary skill sets. Patients are also considered important members of the team. When we collaborate with patients and various healthcare specialists, we can improve the quality of care and achieve the best health outcomes.

Listening practice 1

Listen to the following tracks. Complete the notes below.

◀)) Track 15-1

Situation: _____

Background: _____

Assessment: _____

Recommendation: _____

◀)) Track 15-2

Situation: _____

Background: _____

Assessment: _____

Recommendation: _____

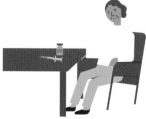

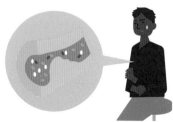

Listening practice 2

Listen to the following conversation between a pharmacist and a physician. Write the missing words and phrases.

🔊 Track 15-3

Pharmacist: Dr. Terry, it's Jones _____.

Physician: Yes, how can I help you?

Pharmacist: I would like to talk to you about one of your patients, John Smith. You _____ the antibiotic levofloxacin. I am concerned about a possible _____ _____ with one of the patient's current medications.

Physician: I see. What _____ is that?

Pharmacist: The patient has a prescription for sotalol from another _____. When combined, sotalol and levofloxacin have a _____ risk for an adverse drug event.

Physician: I was unaware the _____ was taking that medication. Thank you for bringing it to my _____.

Pharmacist: Sure, I am happy to help.

Physician: I am _____ the patient for pneumonia. Is there something else you would _____ that would not have a drug interaction?

Pharmacist: I would _____ using cefuroxime and doxycycline instead to treat the patient's pneumonia. This combination should be _____ without the drug interaction risk.

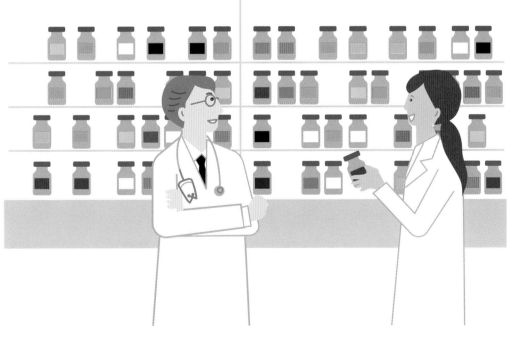

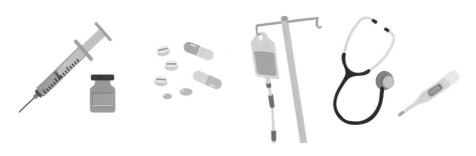 Vocabulary

Below is a list of key vocabulary for this chapter. Translate each word or phrase into your native language.

1. physician _____

2. nurse _____

3. pharmacist _____

4. concise _____

5. dietitian _____

6. social worker _____

7. discipline _____

8. case presentation _____

9. collaborate _____

10. consensus _____

11. compliance _____

12. satisfaction _____

13. comprehensive _____

14. monitoring _____

15. drug interaction _____

16. care plan _____

17. complementary _____

18. colleague _____

19. health outcome _____

20. interprofessional _____

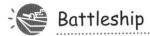

Battleship

1. You have four ships of varying lengths. Place your ships on the map. Ships can be placed vertically and horizontally.
2. Take turns trying to find your partner's ships by stating coordinates, one from the left and one from the top (**Ex** Physician/Compliance). When saying the coordinates, be sure to read the words out loud.
3. For example, if your submarine is at 10-A (Consensus/Compliance) and 10-B (Consensus/Satisfaction), and your partner calls out, "Is there something at Consensus and Compliance?", your partner will get a point because he or she will have found part of your ship.
4. The winner is the one who finds all of his or her partner's ships first or has the most points.

| Battleship | | | | | Cruiser | | | | |
| Carrier | | | | | Submarine | | | | |

My Ships	A Compliance	B Satisfaction	C Comprehensive	D Monitoring	E Drug interaction	F Care plan	G Complementary	H Colleague	I Health outcome	J Interprofessional
1 Physician										
2 Nurse										
3 Pharmacist										
4 Concise										
5 Dietitian										
6 Social worker										
7 Discipline										
8 Presentation										
9 Collaborate										
10 Consensus										

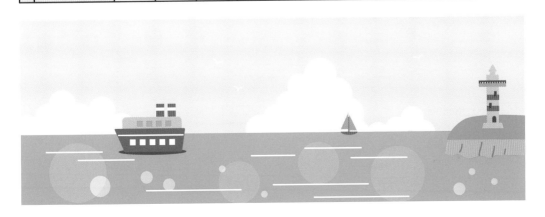

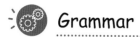 **Grammar**

Conditionals

The conditional is used to express something that might have happened, could happen, or we hope will happen as a result of a condition.

▸ **Conditional sentences have two parts:**

(1) an **if clause** (condition); and

(2) a **main clause** (the result)

> Ex **If you eat pizza every day** (condition), **you will gain weight** (the result).
> Ex **You will gain weight** (the result) **if you eat pizza every day** (condition).

You can put the two parts of the sentence in either order: (1) **condition** + (2) **the result** or (2) **the result** + (1) **condition**. If you put the if clause first, put a comma between the if clause and the main clause.

▸ **There are four types of conditionals:**

(1) **The zero conditional**: Used to express factual and truthful situations and their result.
   This conditional expresses relationships that are always true and never change.
   > Ex If you press this button, the machine turns on.

(2) **The first conditional**: Used to express a possibility and its result.
   This conditional talks about possible situations and shows what you think will happen in those situations.
   > Ex If we work together, we will succeed.

(3) **The second conditional**: Used to express hypothetical situations and their result.
   This conditional talks about an imaginary situation.
   > Ex If we had wings, we would fly. (but we *do not* have wings)

(4) **The third conditional**: Used to express unreal situations and their result.
   This conditional talks about an imagined situation in the past.
   > Ex If I had played, the team would have won. (but I *did not* play)

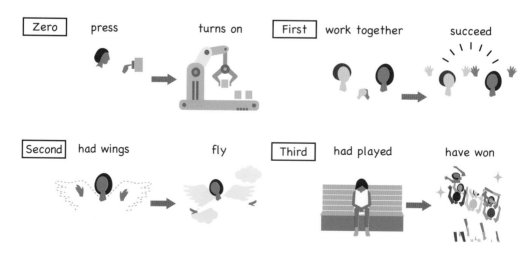

► Conditionals use different tenses:

Type of conditional	If clause	Main clause
(1) Zero	simple present	simple present
(2) First	simple present	simple future
(3) Second	simple past	would + base verb
(4) Third	past perfect	would + have + past participle

💡 Key Points

As the table shows, the if clause almost never uses "will" or "would." Those words, which describe future or hypothetical situations, are the results of the condition; they describe what will happen if the conditions are true, so they go in the main (result) clause.

1 Complete each of the following sentences. Pay special attention to grammatical structure.

1. If you put ice on your injury, the swelling _____ decrease.

2. You _____ pass the exam if you study hard.

3. I would have done my medical training in Europe if I _____ had a lot of money.

4. If I had the ability, I _____ help more people.

5. You _____ recover quickly if you rest.

2 Each of the following sentences contains one or more mistakes. Write the correct versions of the sentences.

1. If we will have more time, we will be able to help more patients.

2. I think his condition would improve if he listens to instructions better.

3. If I see the nurse, I tell her that you have a question.

4. People often feel angry, if they can not control their own health.

5. If the team moves quickly, the mission would have been complete by the end of the day.

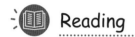 **Reading**

Read the following passage. Answer the questions in the box below.

Team care depends on good communication between healthcare professionals. Communication between different professional groups is called interprofessional communication. This type of communication is different from the one used by healthcare professionals with patients. For example, when talking to patients, it is necessary to speak using simple, non-technical English. Healthcare providers do this so their patients can better understand complicated medical topics. However, this is not the case with interprofessional communication. Instead, professionals from different groups should speak to each other using the language of their profession. When speaking with other healthcare professionals, remember the following points:

✅ The 3Cs
Communication should be **clear**, **comprehensive**, and **concise**. Healthcare professionals are busy and are often "juggling" many tasks and patients at once. Therefore, information must be communicated clearly and concisely to promote understanding and save time. While use of medical jargon is encouraged, it is important to avoid using acronyms and vocabulary that are highly specific to a given discipline.

✅ Collaborative language
Since communication is taking place between two professionals, polite and respectful language should be used. If your words are seen as being rude, it will prevent you from working smoothly with people from other professions or people within your own profession. For example, when making requests, adding phrases like "Would you…" and "Could you…" to the request will be more effective and seem more polite than saying, "Do this." "Would you take Ms. Johnson to Radiology for an MRI?" sounds more polite than "Take Ms. Johnson to Radiology for an MRI." When providing a recommendation, it is better to use phrases like "I suggest…" and "I recommend…" instead of "You should…".

✅ Cultural competency
Awareness of cultural differences is important not only for dealing with patients but also for interacting with colleagues and other healthcare professionals. That is because, for a team to function effectively, all members of the team must feel mutual respect from other members of the team. Feelings of discrimination or disrespect can cause members of the team to not want to cooperate or do their best.

---

1. What is interprofessional communication?
2. How is interprofessional communication different from communication between healthcare professionals and patients?
3. What are the 3Cs, and how do they help with interprofessional communication?
4. How would you define collaborative communication?
5. Why is cultural competency important in interprofessional communication?

Speaking & writing

Look at the following questions. Write down your opinion in response to each question. Share your opinions with the class, in small groups, or with your teacher.

1. What challenges have you faced while working in a group? How did you solve them?
2. What problems can occur if the team does not communicate effectively? Give examples.

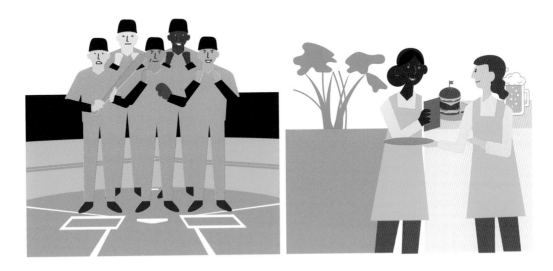

 ## What do you think?

Look at the following questions. Write down your opinion in response to each question. Share your opinions with the class, in small groups, or with your teacher.

1. Who do you think is the most important member of the healthcare team? Why?
2. Can you think of any other ways to improve team-based communication?
3. How do you feel about working with a team to treat patients? Are there any drawbacks?

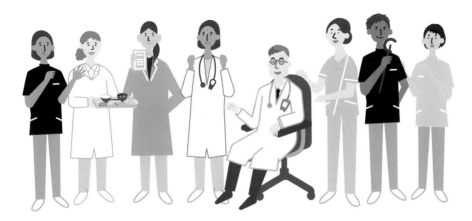

Language corner

Use SBAR (Situation, Background, Assessment, and Recommendation) when communicating information about patients with your teammates and during case presentations.

✅ Situation

A brief statement of the problem. It is usually a description of the patient's chief complaint.

> **Useful phrases**
> Mr. Smith is a 40-year-old male presenting with a severe headache.

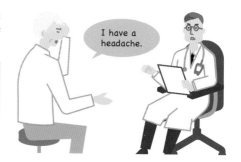

✅ Background

Important information that is related to the situation. This information may include past medical history and medication history.

> **Useful phrases**
> Mr. Smith has had a headache for a week. He also visited our clinic a month ago with the same symptoms.

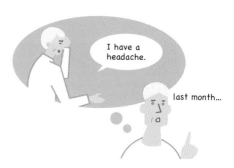

✅ Assessment

Assessing the problem based on current medical findings.

> **Useful phrases**
> Based on the location and description of the headache, it may be a migraine, or it could be something more serious.

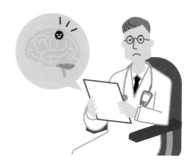

✅ Recommendation

Giving precise information on what needs to be done moving forward.

> **Useful phrases**
> I suggest the patient receive an MRI to rule out brain tumor.

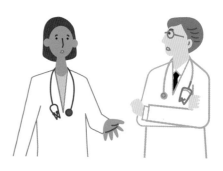

Team care in action

Traditionally, patients with chronic diseases, such as diabetes, are managed by a physician. The Santa Clara Valley Medical Center in California, USA, wanted to try a different approach. They decided to start an interprofessional clinic. In this clinic, a team of healthcare professionals collaborate to treat patients.

For example, if a patient is having nutrition problems, a dietitian is consulted. Pharmacists educate the patients about their medicine. Furthermore, if a patient needs support in their daily lives, social workers are there to help. Physicians are still very important in the interprofessional clinic. However, here they do not need to make decisions alone. After all the team members discuss the patient and offer recommendations, the team reaches a consensus on the best care plan for the patient.

This team-based approach has been very effective and is well liked by the patients. As a result, the Santa Clara Valley Medical Center interprofessional clinic has been able to improve patient health outcomes and patient satisfaction. This approach is now being used in many medical facilities around the world.

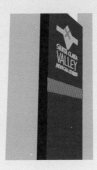

 # Homework

Find three people with different healthcare specialties on campus or in your community. Please interview them and collect the following information:

1. Specialty
2. Educational background
3. General expertise
4. Work responsibilities
5. Experience with team-based care

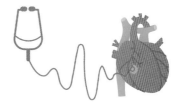

15

Team care

重要語句一覧

Vocabulary list

医療系学生のためのつたわる英語 ［Web音声付］
―English Communication Competency for Future Healthcare Professionals

2022年2月25日　発行	監修者　代田浩之
	編集者　並木有希, Marcellus Nealy,
	Tom Kain
	発行者　小立健太
	発行所　株式会社 南 江 堂

〒113-8410　東京都文京区本郷三丁目42番6号
☎(出版)03-3811-7236　(営業)03-3811-7239
ホームページ https://www.nankodo.co.jp/
印刷・製本 シナノ書籍印刷
組版・デザイン アスラン編集スタジオ

© Nankodo Co., Ltd., 2022

定価は表紙に表示してあります.
落丁・乱丁の場合はお取り替えいたします.
ご意見・お問い合わせはホームページまでお寄せください.

Printed and Bound in Japan
ISBN 978-4-524-22813-3